# Cannabis Dessert Cookbook

## 50 Wicked Good Marijuana Sweet Recipes

**George Green**

ISBN: 9798584835026

# CONTENTS

# INTRODUCTION

The joy and satisfaction of weed-infused edibles is something we're all fond of. But the world of weed edibles has a lot more to offer to make the best use of recreational cannabis. Weed desserts? Who doesn't need an excuse to make one of them? With THC-infused desserts, you can satisfy your sweet tooth and put an end to those sweet cravings while also experiencing that exclusive cannabis buzz.

Cannabis desserts give you a relaxing, fulfilling, and long-lasting experience. More importantly, when you consume marijuana in its edible form, it passes through your liver, making it a healthier option as compared to vaping or smoking. Canna-butter is the building block for most weed-infused desserts; canna-oil is another foundational ingredient used in many dessert recipes.

Making yourself a perfect dessert is a worthwhile reward for the trouble of finding or growing marijuana. Brownies, muffins, and cookies are some of the classic cannabis desserts that are popular worldwide. It's time to give your kitchen a high time with those world-famous—or should we say, world-infamous—desserts and make the best of your day. Here we have got some exciting dessert recipes for you to try out and prove yourself to be a true weed aficionado. Introduce your best bud to these amazing dessert recipes and dive into the incredible world of weed desserts.

With the right use of recreational marijuana, you can prepare plenty of scrumptious, creative desserts in your kitchen. From cakes to pies and brownies to cookies, this cookbook presents a diverse range of cannabis desserts so you can enjoy all your mouthwatering cannabis dessert favorites anytime you like. Master the art of preparing marijuana desserts at home as you explore the ultimate collection of 60 succulent marijuana dessert recipes to get you going. The recipes are easy to prepare using cannabis-infused butter and cannabis-infused oil. With these simple to follow instructions, you can now prepare a wide range of desserts such as brownies, sweet breads, cupcakes, pies, bars, muffins, cakes, cookies, truffles, fudge and so on.

Before we dig into the recipes, let's get familiar with the world of cannabis and the principles of cooking with cannabis.

# Welcome to the World of Cannabis

The cannabis plant contains many cannabinoid compounds, but the two most important ones are cannabidiol (CBD) and tetrahydrocannabinol (THC).

CBD is non-psychoactive, meaning that it does not deliver that "high" effect, but scientific experiments and studies have confirmed that it has a wide variety of medical uses. CBD helps to regulate the body's state of balance or "homeostasis". In short, it positively affects appetite, sleep, immune response, mood, and hormone regulation.

THC, on the other hand, does deliver that "high" effect. THC attaches to the cannabinoid receptors in the brain to cause psychological effects. It also influences certain areas of the brain that are responsible for pleasure, memory, and movement.

Taken together, THC and CBD work synergistically to optimize each other's curative properties. CBD activates the anti-cancer and analgesic properties of THC while reducing its psychoactivity. CBD can also ease rapid heartbeat, anxiety, and other adverse side effects caused by taking THC in large dosages.

Some pharmaceutical companies have successfully created cannabis-based drugs to treat certain health conditions and disorders. These drugs contain more CBD or THC according to their purpose. Cannabis is also being sold commercially in various forms such as tinctures, capsules, sprays, and topical creams.

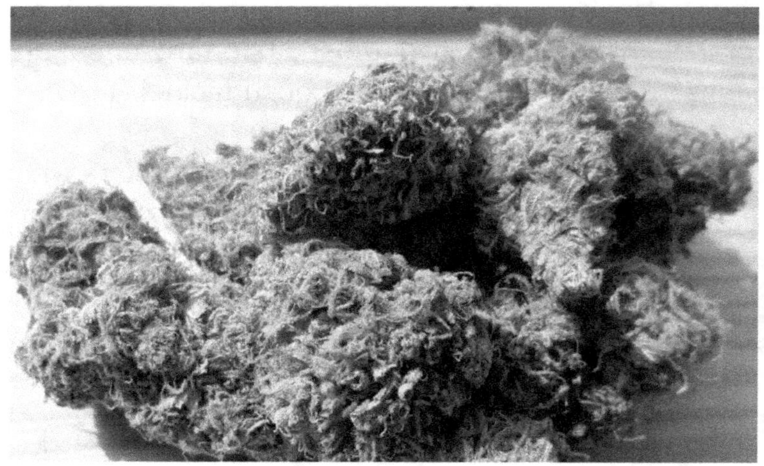

# Cannabis Medicinal Properties

Much research and many scientific studies, including a review published by the *British Journal of Pharmacology* in 2013, have discussed the possible medicinal properties of CBD. Most of these studies have been conducted on animals; only a few of them included human subjects.

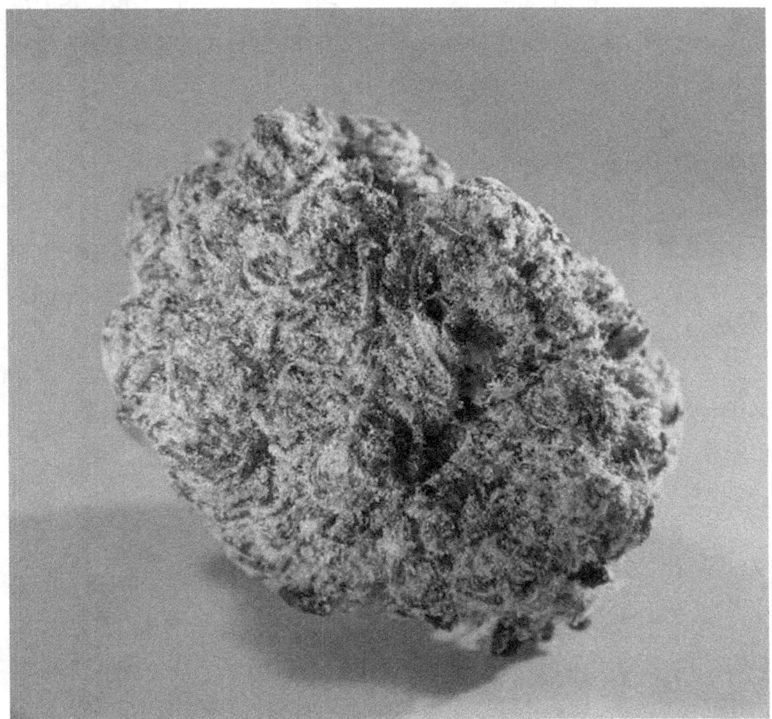

The studies concluded that the use of cannabis may deliver the following medicinal effects:

**Anti-inflammatory**

Cannabis minimizes inflammation to prevent inflammatory disorders, including glaucoma. According to a review published by the National Eye Institute based in Bethesda, Maryland, cannabis aids in minimizing the pressure within the eyeball and thus helps control the symptoms of glaucoma, an eye condition marked by increased pressure within the eyeball, which leads to gradual loss of vision. Cannabis may decrease the pressure in the eye and prevent or delay vision loss.

**Respiratory Effects**

A study published in the *Journal of the American Medical Association* in 2012 suggested that smoking cannabis does not hamper the function of the lungs. In fact, smoking cannabis may improve lung capacity.

**Antipsychotic and Antidepressant**

Cannabis fights various psychosis disorders, as well as the symptoms of depression and anxiety.

There has been much scientific research analyzing the effects of medical cannabis in controlling the symptoms of mental disorders such as anxiety, major depression, bipolar disorder, mania, panic disorder, schizophrenia, and other forms of psychosis.

A study conducted in 2006 by the *Molecular Pharmaceutics Journal* stated that cannabis can be effective in controlling the progression of Alzheimer's disease.

## Anticonvulsant

In the mid-19th century, the *United States Pharmacopeia* described cannabis tincture as a valid treatment for pediatric epilepsy. Later studies indicated that the anticonvulsant properties of the cannabis plant may help minimize the frequency and intensity of temporal and parietal lobe seizures.

## Antidiabetic

Studies have also found that cannabis positively affects fasting insulin and insulin resistance. Additional benefits listed by the American Alliance for Medical Cannabis (2005) include suggestions that it is a vasodilator and an antispasmodic agent, and that it relieves the symptoms of Restless Leg Syndrome (RLS) and neuropathic pain.

## Antiemetic and Antioxidant

Cannabis protects against cell damage and oxidation, thereby preventing neurodegenerative diseases.

Cannabis consumption may help in relieving or controlling nausea and vomiting.

**Anticancer/Anti-tumoral**
Research from the California Pacific Medical Center appearing in the *Molecular Cancer Therapeutics* journal in 2007 reported that CBD may be effective in preventing the spread of cancer by shutting down a gene known as Id-This gene activates cancer cells and prompts them to spread throughout the body.

**Multiple Sclerosis**
Multiple sclerosis leads to many painful symptoms. Medical cannabis can be an effective option to minimize pain and muscle spasms.

**Pain Relief**
One of the most common uses of medical cannabis is for pain relief. THC may relieve pain by stimulating the pathways within the central nervous system that block the pain signals from reaching the brain.

**Asthma**
CBD may deliver potent immunosuppressive and anti-inflammatory effects that are extremely helpful in controlling the symptoms of asthma. THC may also help in calming asthma attacks.

# Creative Cooking with Cannabis

Whether you are an experienced smoker, a recreational user, or just a cannabis enthusiast, there are many creative ways to give your taste buds a hint of cannabis.

Cannabis recipes offer a little medicated flavor and contain only a slight hint of cannabis. It takes 1–2 hours to feel the effects of ingested cannabis as THC enters the blood through the digestive system.

# Cooking with Already Been Vaped (ABV) Cannabis

AVB (Already Vaped Bud), also popularly known as Already Been Vaped (ABV), is the plant matter that remains after cannabis is vaporized. Vaporizing is a different way of inhaling cannabis, similar to smoking. The two most common methods of preparing ABV are:

**1) Manual Hot Water Technique**
This involves submerging cannabis completely in a pot of hot water. Let the cannabis rest in the hot water for 30–45 minutes. Discard the water and preserve the cannabis. Heat more water in a separate pot and

then add it to the cannabis pot. Again let it rest for 30–45 minutes. Repeat until the discarded water does not smell like cannabis. Dry out the cannabis at room temperature or in sunlight.

## 2) Cannabis Vaporizing Machine

This involves heating cannabis at 300–400°F using a cannabis vaporizing machine. When heated at these temperatures, cannabis releases the psychoactive compound THC. Vaporizing is increasing in popularity as the technique prevents the inhalation of unwanted gases and tars that are released when smoking cannabis. These machines are different than water pipes.

Vaped cannabis is dark brown in color and has a subtle, distinct aroma in comparison to fresh cannabis buds. Many people simply discard ABV because they believe that they have already extracted all its essence and mood-enhancing benefits. However, you can still get more out of your ABV.

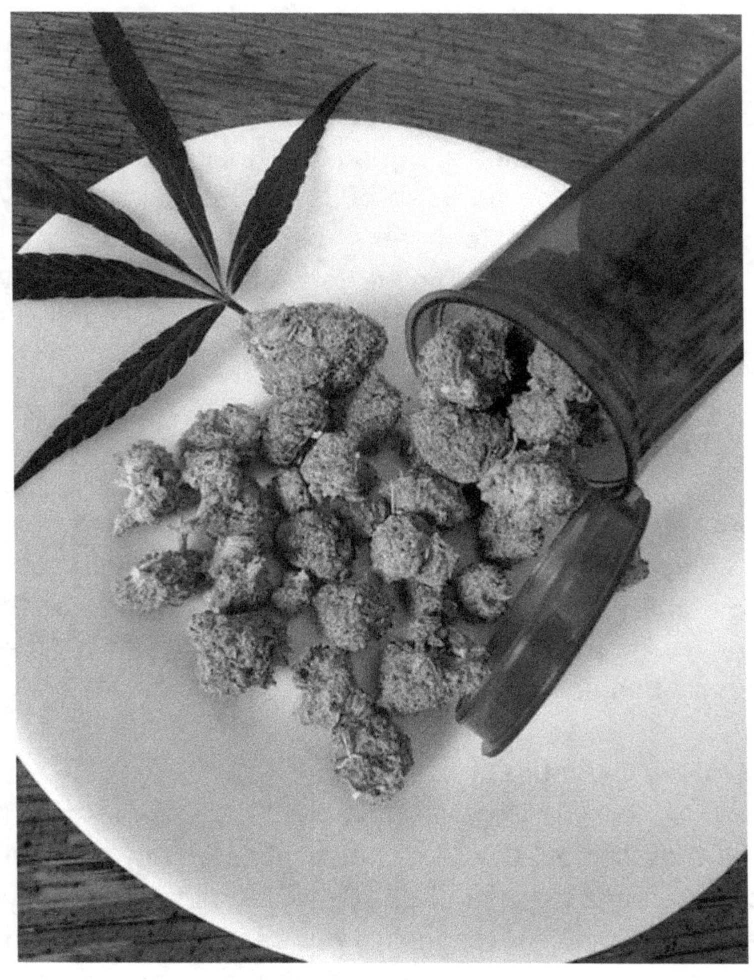

Decarboxylation (explained in the next section) is the chemical process that happens when cannabis gives up a carbon molecule, usually through heating. Until this happens, the plant has very little effect on people. As ABV has already been de-carbed, one can use it for several different purposes:

## 1) Smoking

You can smoke cannabis that has already been vaped, although not a lot of cannabis users do this. ABV does not taste very good and does not deliver as much stimulation as fresh buds do. People generally prefer vaporizing cannabis because it does not combust the herb, and obviously smoking ABV totally defeats this purpose. However, you can still get slight stimulation from smoking ABV.

## 2) Direct Approach

If you prefer ingesting the plant material directly, you can sprinkle ABV buds (only a fraction of an ounce) onto your pizzas, sandwiches and pastas, or into your smoothies and drinks. ABV tastes very similar to fresh buds with almost the same aroma, but with a little more "toasted" flavor.

## 3) ABV Coconut Oil

This works great for your favorite pastas, snacks and salad dressings. Over low heat, mix a pint of coconut oil and half an ounce of ABV in a saucepan until they are incorporated. Optionally, you can use soy lecithin to bind everything together. Strain the oil and store it in the refrigerator for later use.

## 4) Canna-butter

Canna-butter is quite popular and has been used in hundreds of cannabis-infused recipes. Use ABV and butter in a 1:1 ratio to make canna-butter. The quantity of water needed depends on the volume of the ingredients; use adequate water to cover the ingredients in a saucepan.

# Why it is Important to Decarboxylate Cannabis

In its raw form, the cannabis plant is non-psychoactive. It only becomes psychoactive when the buds dry out, when they age, or when they are heated. Heating activates more psychoactive compounds than aging. In order to release the maximum potential of the plant's psychoactive compounds, the decarboxylating or "decarbing" process must be completed.

**Decarboxylation Process**
1. Preheat oven to 240°F.
2. Break cannabis buds and flowers into smaller bits using your hands.
3. Arrange the pieces in a single layer on a medium-sized baking pan lined with parchment paper.
4. The cannabis should cover the pan completely so that there is no empty space on the sheet.
5. Bake the buds for 35–40 minutes. Stir two or three times in between for even toasting.

6. After the buds dry out and darken, remove the pan from the oven and let it cool for 20–25 minutes. The texture should be crumbly.
7. In a food processor, process the buds until they are coarsely ground. Be careful you do not over-process and turn the cannabis into powder.
8. Store in an airtight glass container.
9. Follow the same process for decarbing kief and stems. (Dried resin buds, collected from cannabis plant leaves, are used to make kief. These buds can be ground to make fine powder, which is known as "kief".)

# Decarboxylated Cannabis-Infused Oil

Decarboxylated cannabis (prepared as above) is used to make cannabis-infused oil. Pick an oil that has a high fat content and is made from an unmodified, natural crop. Oils with low heating points are best, as they preserve the original taste of the oil after the cannabis flavor is infused. Below are some recommended oils to use for cannabis infusion:

**1) Olive Oil**
Olive oil is incredibly healthy, natural, and flavorful. It is perfectly suited for salad dressings, flatbread pizza, pastas, or as a dip to use with your favorite bread.

Use high-quality extra virgin olive oil made from natural, real olives and not the colored or repackaged versions of vegetable oils.

**2) Coconut Oil**
Coconut oil is one of the most recommended choices for preparing cannabis-infused oil because it contains the highest saturated fat content. It thus absorbs more cannabinoids than other oils. It also has a better shelf life when processed or heated.

# Making Canna-butter or Cannabis Butter at Home

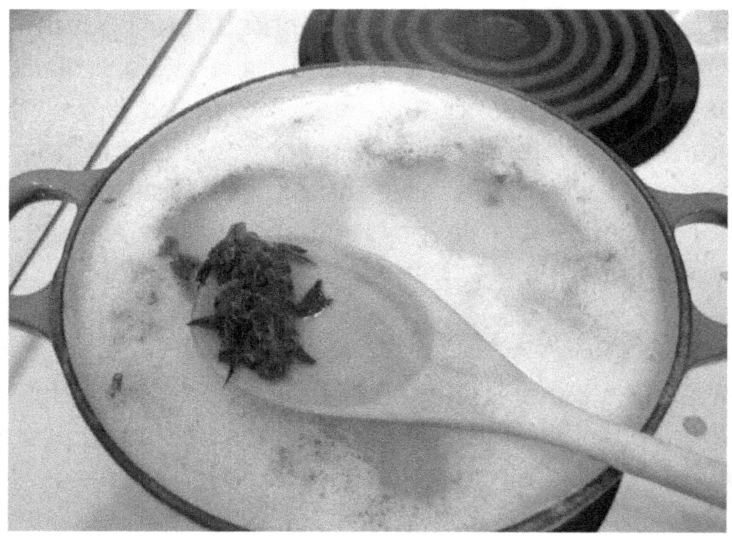

### Ingredients

1 cup water

1 pound unsalted butter

1 ounce cannabis, coarsely ground

### Directions

1. Place the unsalted butter and water in a stockpot or saucepan.
2. Gradually warm the pot over low heat.
3. Let the butter melt and bring it to a simmer to completely melt the butter into the water.
4. Stir the flower into the mixture.

5. Simmer for 2½–3 hours, stirring occasionally. Do not let the mixture boil.
6. Pour the mixture into a glass container with a tight-fitting lid.
7. Use a piece of cheesecloth or a fine metal strainer to filter out the plant material from the prepared mix.
8. Squeeze the cheesecloth to extract all the liquid. Discard the remaining plant material.
9. Cool for 10–15 minutes.
10. Cover and store the canna-butter in the refrigerator for 10–12 hours to harden.
11. The hardened butter will separate from the water so you can easily take it out and use it in your recipes.
12. Discard the remaining water.
13. Store the canna-butter at room temperature if you will use it soon.
14. You can also store it in the freezer for later use. The butter stays good for 2–3 months when stored in a freezer. When you're ready to use it, take it out and let it thaw at room temperature for 15–20 minutes before using. (There is no need to warm it up in a microwave or oven.)

# Making Cannabis Oil at Home

**Ingredients**

1⅖ ounces decarboxylated cannabis
2 cups unrefined coconut oil

**Directions**

1. Mix the coconut oil and cannabis in a saucepan. Gradually warm it over low heat.
2. Simmer the mixture for 50–60 minutes, stirring occasionally. Do not cover the pan.
3. Place a metal strainer lined with cheesecloth over a bowl to filter out the cannabis particles.
4. Pour the mixture into the strainer and allow it to drip for about 60–75 minutes.
5. Wrap the plant material in the cheesecloth and squeeze out any leftover liquid. Discard the solids.
6. Cool the liquid mixture in a glass container for 10–15 minutes and allow it to solidify.
7. Cover the container and place it in the refrigerator. The oil is usually good for up to 10–12 months.

# Making Canna-cream or Canna-milk at Home

### *Ingredients*

½ ounce decarboxylated cannabis, finely crumbled
1¼ cups of your choice of heavy whipping cream, whole milk, almond milk or coconut milk

### *Directions*

1. Fill a deep saucepan with water and simmer it.
2. Fold up a kitchen towel and place it in the bottom of the saucepan.
3. Add the milk and crumbled cannabis to a wide mouth 16-ounce canning jar such as a Mason jar. Close the lid and place the jar in the simmering water over the folded towel. The water should cover tree quarter of the jar.
4. Simmer for 80–90 minutes, topping up the water as needed.
5. Take the jar out of the water every 20 minutes with tongs and pot holders and carefully open the lid to stir the milk with a wooden spoon and release pressure.
6. Cool down completely and store in an airtight container in your fridge up to 3–5 days.

# Being Safe while Infusing

- If possible, infuse oils outside in the open air to minimize the risk of fire or explosion. If you are inside, open the windows and start a fan for better air circulation.
- If you have a respiratory condition or sensitive lungs, use a facemask.
- Make sure that you are using proper equipment. While preparing an infusion that involves solvents, a double boiler pot and pan setup is better, with the solvent pan being on top of the water pot, and not directly on the heating element of the stove. Follow this precaution with both gas and electric stoves. Always wear a face mask when working with solvents.
- To avoid unexpected hazards, prepare canna infusion oil when there are minimum distractions and you're not in a hurry.
- Be more alert when preparing infusion oil or butter on a gas stove. Avoid placing the solvent pan near the stove when the flame is on, as it can catch fire.
- Once you're finished making canna oil or butter, be sure to turn off the oven, the stove and any other open flame heating element.
- Store your oils and edibles in child-resistant containers in a dry place that is difficult for children and pets to reach. Accidental

ingestion of cannabis-infused oil by children
and pets may lead to many health issues.

Now we are ready to dig in right and find that perfect
sweet combination to enjoy recreational marijuana
and delicious desserts at the same time.

# BREAD AND BROWNIES

## Pumpkin Bread

*Serves about 14 slices*
*Preparation time: 10 minutes*
*Cooking time: 40 minutes*

### Ingredients

½ teaspoon baking powder
1 teaspoon baking soda
¾ cup wheat flour
⅔ cup all-purpose flour
1 teaspoon ground cinnamon
½ teaspoon nutmeg
¼ teaspoon salt
½ cup packed brown sugar
⅓ cup canna-oil
1 cup pumpkin puree
⅓ cup honey
2 eggs

### Directions

1. Preheat the oven to 350°F (175°C). Grease an 8×4-inch loaf pan with some butter or cooking spray.
2. Mix the baking soda, baking powder, nutmeg, cinnamon, flours and salt together in a mixing bowl.

3.  In another bowl, beat the eggs. Add the sugar, canna-oil, pumpkin puree and honey. Mix well.
4.  Combine the two mixtures and mix until smooth and without visible lumps.
5.  Add the batter to the loaf pan. Smooth the surface with a spatula or spoon.
6.  Bake for 40 minutes until the top turns golden brown. Check by inserting a toothpick; if it doesn't come out clean, bake for a few more minutes and repeat.
7.  Remove from oven and let cool completely on a wire rack.
8.  Slice and serve.

***Nutrition (per serving)***

Calories 116

Carbs 21g, Fat 1g, Protein 2g, Sodium 134mg

# Banana Bread

*Serves 15*
*Preparation time: 10 minutes*
*Cooking time: 1 hour*

**Ingredients**
1 cup sugar
½ cup canna-butter, melted
2 eggs
1 teaspoon vanilla extract
½ cup sour cream
½ cup walnuts, chopped
2 bananas, peeled and sliced
1½ cups all-purpose flour
1 teaspoon baking soda
½ teaspoon salt

**Directions**
1. Preheat the oven to 350°F (175°C). Grease an 8×5-inch loaf pan with some butter or cooking spray.
2. In a mixing bowl, beat the butter and sugar until fluffy. Add the eggs and vanilla. Mix well.
3. Mix in the sour cream, walnuts and bananas.
4. Mix the flour, baking soda and salt together in a mixing bowl.
5. Combine the two mixtures and mix until smooth and without visible lumps.
6. Add the batter to the loaf pan. Smooth the surface with a spatula or spoon.

7. Bake for 1 hour until the top turns golden brown. Check by inserting a toothpick; if it doesn't come out clean, bake for a few more minutes and repeat.
8. Remove from oven and let cool completely on a wire rack.
9. Slice and serve.

**Nutrition (per serving)**
Calories 215
Carbs 27g, Fat 11g, Protein 3g, Sodium 220mg

# Zucchini Bread

*Serves 28–32 slices*
*Preparation time: 10–15 minutes*
*Cooking time: 1 hour*

**Ingredients**

1 teaspoon baking soda
½ teaspoon baking powder
2½ teaspoons cinnamon
1 teaspoon ground nutmeg
3 cups flour
1 cup canna-butter, melted
1¾ cups sugar
2 teaspoons vanilla extract
3 eggs
2 cups zucchini, grated
1 cup chopped pecans

**Directions**

1. Preheat the oven to 325°F (160°C). Grease two 8×4-inch loaf pans with some butter or cooking spray.
2. Mix together the baking soda, baking powder, nutmeg, cinnamon, flour and salt.
3. In a mixing bowl, beat the butter and sugar until fluffy. Add the eggs, one at a time, and vanilla. Mix well.
4. Combine the two mixtures and mix until smooth and without visible lumps.
5. Mix in the zucchini and pecans.

6.  Add the batter to the loaf pans. Smooth the surface with a spatula or spoon.
7.  Bake for 1 hour until the top turns golden brown. Check by inserting a toothpick; if it doesn't come out clean, bake for a few more minutes and repeat.
8.  Remove from oven and let cool completely on a wire rack.
9.  Slice and serve.

**Nutrition (per serving)**

Calories 162

Carbs 20g, Fat 8g, Protein 2g, Sodium 56mg

# Chocolate Chip Brownies

*Serves 8-9*
*Preparation time: 10 minutes*
*Cooking time: 30 minutes*

### Ingredients

¾ cup all-purpose flour

½ cup unsweetened cocoa powder

½ teaspoon salt

¼ teaspoon baking powder

½ cup canna-butter or canna-oil

1 cup white sugar

¼ cup brown sugar

2 large eggs

1 teaspoon vanilla extract

Toppings: Nuts, chocolate chips, sea salt (optional)

¼ teaspoon vegetable shortening

### Directions

1. Preheat the oven to 350°F (175°C). Grease an 8×8-inch baking pan with some butter or cooking spray.
2. Mix the dry ingredients together in a mixing bowl.
3. In another mixing bowl, beat the canna-butter/canna-oil and sugar until fluffy. Add the eggs, one at a time, and vanilla. Mix well.
4. Combine the two mixtures and mix until smooth and without visible lumps.
5. Add the batter to the pan and smooth the surface with a spatula or spoon.

6. Bake for 25–30 minutes until golden brown.
7. Check by inserting a toothpick. For brownies it won't necessarily come out clean, but what's on it shouldn't be batter-like. If it is, bake for a few more minutes and repeat.
8. Remove from oven and let cool for 5–10 minutes on a wire rack.
9. Slice into squares and serve warm.

**Nutrition (per serving)**
Calories 240
Carbs 19g, Fat 17g, Protein 4g, Sodium 212mg

# **Marshmallow Brownies**

*Serves 10 pieces*
*Preparation time: 10 minutes*
*Cooking time: 15-20 minutes*

**Ingredients**
2 large eggs
1 teaspoon vanilla extract
¼ teaspoon salt
¼ teaspoon baking powder
1 cup brown sugar
½ cup whole wheat baking flour or all-purpose flour
¼ cup canna-butter
¼ cup vegetable oil
⅓ cup cocoa powder
4 graham crackers, crumbled
8 ounces milk chocolate, chopped
1 cup mini marshmallows

**Directions**
1. Preheat the oven to 350°F (175°C). Line a medium baking pan with parchment paper.
2. In another bowl, beat the eggs. Add the vanilla, salt, baking powder and brown sugar. Mix well.
3. Mix together the flour, canna-butter, vegetable oil and cocoa powder.
4. Combine the two mixtures and mix until smooth and without visible lumps.

5. Add the batter to the pan and smooth the surface with a spatula or spoon. Bake for 15 minutes.
6. Meanwhile, combine the graham crackers, milk chocolate and marshmallows.
7. Top the brownies with the marshmallow mixture.
8. Bake for 15–20 minutes more until golden brown. Check by inserting a toothpick. For brownies it won't necessarily come out clean, but what's on it shouldn't be batter-like. If it is, bake for a few more minutes and repeat.
9. Remove from oven and let cool for 5–10 minutes on a wire rack.
10. Slice into squares and serve warm.

**Nutrition (per serving)**
Calories 269
Carbs 36g, Fat 13g, Protein 4g, Sodium 128mg

# Macadamia Choco Brownies

*Serves Makes 12 brownies*
*Preparation time: 8-10 minutes*
*Baking time: 30 minutes*


**Ingredients**
¾ cup all-purpose flour
3 eggs
½ teaspoon vanilla extract
2 tablespoons cocoa powder
¾ teaspoon salt
⅓ cup coconut oil
¼ cup cannabis coconut oil
4½ ounces unsweetened chocolate
1 cup packed brown sugar
¾ cup chopped pecans, macadamia nuts, or almonds
(optional)
Unsalted butter, melted to grease


**Directions**
1.  Preheat oven to 350°F or 176°C. Line an 8×8 baking pan with aluminum foil and grease with some cooking spray.
2.  Mix the flour, cocoa powder and salt in a mixing bowl.
3.  To a medium skillet or saucepan, add both the oils and heat over medium heat.
4.  Add the chocolate and cook until it melts completely.
5.  Set aside to cool for 5 minutes.

6.  Mix the brown sugar in with the melted chocolate.
7.  Beat the eggs in a bowl and mix in the vanilla extract. Combine well.
8.  Add in the flour mix and combine well; mix in the nuts.
9.  Add the batter into the prepared pan and bake for 25–30 minutes, or until a toothpick comes out clean.
10. Take out and let cool; slice and serve.

**Nutrition (per slice)**
Calories 268
Carbs 24.6g, Fat 16.8g, Protein 3.6g, Sodium 224mg

# Triple Delight Brownies

*Serves 18 squares*
*Preparation time: 10 minutes*
*Cooking time: 25 minutes*

### Ingredients

3 sticks unsalted butter

3 tablespoons canna-butter

6 eggs, cold

1¾ cups brown sugar

1 tablespoon vanilla extract

1½ cups all-purpose or whole wheat baking flour

1 teaspoon salt

12 ounces bittersweet chocolate

⅛ cup unsweetened cocoa powder

½ cup chocolate chips

½ cup macadamia nuts (optional)

### Directions

1. Preheat the oven to 350°F (175°C). Line an 8×8-inch baking pan with parchment paper.
2. Melt the canna-butter and butter over medium heat in a medium saucepan or skillet.
3. Add the chocolate and stir-cook until completely melted. Let cool for a few minutes.
4. In another bowl, beat the eggs. Add the sugar and vanilla. Mix well.
5. Mix in the chocolate mixture.
6. Mix the salt, cocoa powder and flour together in a mixing bowl.

7.    Combine the two mixtures and mix until
      smooth and with no visible lumps.
8.    Mix in the chocolate chips.
9.    Add the batter to the pan and smooth the
      surface with a spatula or spoon.
10.   Bake for 25 minutes until golden brown.
      Check by inserting a toothpick. For brownies
      it won't necessarily come out clean, but
      what's on it shouldn't be batter-like. If it is,
      bake for a few more minutes and repeat.
11.   Remove from oven and let cool for 5–10
      minutes on a wire rack.
12.   Slice into squares and serve warm.

***Nutrition (per serving)***
Calories 303
Carbs 28g, Fat 17g, Protein 5g, Sodium 341mg

# Coconut Brownies

*Serves 16 pieces*
*Preparation time: 10 minutes*
*Cooking time: 20–25 minutes*

### Ingredients

2 tablespoons canna-butter

6 tablespoons unsalted butter

1 cup dark brown sugar

1 large egg, cold

1½ teaspoons vanilla extract

⅛ teaspoon salt

1 cup whole wheat or all-purpose flour

½ cup shredded coconut

½ cup toasted nuts (optional)

### Directions:

1. Preheat the oven to 350°F (175°C). Line an 8×8-inch baking pan with parchment paper.
2. In a mixing bowl, beat the butter, canna-butter and sugar until fluffy. Add the egg and vanilla. Mix well.
3. Add the flour and salt and combine well.
4. Mix in the shredded coconut and toasted nuts. Whisk to make a thick batter.
5. Add the batter to the pan and smooth the surface with a spatula or spoon.
6. Bake for 20–25 minutes until golden brown. Check by inserting a toothpick. For brownies it won't necessarily come out clean, but what's

on it shouldn't be batter-like. If it is, bake for a few more minutes and repeat.
7.  Remove from oven and let cool for 5–10 minutes on a wire rack.
8.  Slice into squares and serve warm.

**Nutrition (per serving)**
Calories 281
Carbs 32g, Fat 14g, Protein 3g, Sodium 88mg

# Mint Buttercream Brownies

*Serves 12 - Preparation time: 20–25 minutes*
*Cooking time: 30 minutes*

### Ingredients
½ cup canna-butter
4 ounces semi-sweet chocolate, chopped
¾ cup white sugar
¼ cup packed brown sugar
2 large eggs
½ teaspoon peppermint extract
⅓ cup all-purpose flour
⅛ cup cocoa powder
¼ teaspoon salt

Buttercream
⅓ cup unsalted butter
1 cup confectioners' sugar
1 tablespoon cream or milk
¾ teaspoon peppermint extract
Few drops of green food coloring

Glaze
⅓ cup unsalted butter
1 cup chocolate chips

### Directions
1. Preheat the oven to 350°F (175°C). Line an 8×8-inch baking pan with parchment paper and grease it with some butter or cooking spray.

2.  Melt the chocolate and canna-butter over medium heat in a saucepan until smooth.
3.  Let cool for 5–10 minutes.
4.  Mix in both of the sugars until completely dissolved. Mix in the beaten egg and mint extract.
5.  Mix together the flour, salt and cocoa powder.
6.  Combine the two mixtures and mix until smooth and without visible lumps.
7.  Bake for 25–30 minutes until golden brown. Check by inserting a toothpick. For brownies it won't necessarily come out clean, but what's on it shouldn't be batter-like. If it is, bake for a few more minutes and repeat.
8.  Remove from oven and let cool for 5–10 minutes on a wire rack.

Cream Layer
1.  In a mixing bowl, beat the butter and sugar until fluffy. Add the milk and food coloring. Mix well.
2.  Spread the mixture over the baked brownie.
3.  Refrigerate for 1–2 hours.

Glaze
1.  Melt the butter and chocolate chips over medium-low heat in a medium saucepan or skillet.
2.  Let cool for a few minutes.
3.  Pour the glaze over the brownies and spread to make an even layer.
4.  Refrigerate for another hour.
5.  Slice into squares and serve.

**Nutrition (per serving)**

Calories 419

Carbs 41g, Fat 22g, Protein 7g, Sodium 106mg

# CUPCAKES, PIES, AND BARS

## Bacon Spice Cupcakes

*Serves 12*
*Preparation time: 10 minutes*
*Cooking time: 25 minutes*

### Ingredients
1½ teaspoons baking powder
1½ cups all-purpose flour
1 cup sugar
1 teaspoon ground cinnamon
½ teaspoon ground allspice
¼ teaspoon grated nutmeg
½ teaspoon salt
½ cup canna-butter, softened
½ cup sour cream
2 large eggs
½ teaspoon maple extract
4 slices bacon, cut into 12 pieces

Topping
¼ cup all-purpose flour
¼ cup sugar
2½ tablespoons unsalted butter, chilled and cut into ½-inch pieces
½ teaspoon ground cinnamon
¼ cup pecans, chopped

### *Directions*

1. Preheat the oven to 350°F (175°C). Line a 12-cup muffin or cupcake pan with paper liners.
2. To make the topping, mix the flour, sugar, butter, cinnamon and pecans together in a mixing bowl. Set aside.
3. To make the batter, mix the baking powder, flour, sugar, cinnamon, allspice, nutmeg and salt together in a mixing bowl.
4. In another mixing bowl, beat the butter and cream until fluffy. Add the eggs, one at a time. Mix well.
5. Mix in the maple extract.
6. Combine the two mixtures and mix until smooth and without visible lumps.
7. Evenly distribute the batter among the cups. Sprinkle the topping mixture evenly on top. Check by inserting a toothpick; if it doesn't come out clean, bake for a few more minutes and repeat.
8. Bake for 20–25 minutes until golden brown. Check by inserting a toothpick; if it doesn't come out clean, bake for a few more minutes and repeat.
9. Leave the pan in the oven for 5 minutes to cool slightly.
10. Remove from oven and let cool on a wire rack for 10–15 minutes.
11. Place one bacon piece over each cupcake and press. Serve warm.

### *Nutrition (per serving)*

Calories 223

Carbs 32g, Fat 8g, Protein 4g, Sodium 197mg

# Coffee Ganache Cupcakes

*Serves 8-10 cupcakes*
*Preparation time: 10 minutes*
*Cooking time: 30 minutes*

### Ingredients
¼ cup canna-butter

1 cup sugar

4 large eggs, room temperature

2 cups chocolate syrup

1 tablespoon vanilla extract

1 cup all-purpose flour

1 teaspoon instant coffee granules

Ganache

½ cup heavy cream

½ pound semisweet chocolate morsels

½ teaspoon instant coffee

### Directions
1. Preheat the oven to 325°F (160°C). Line a 12-cup muffin or cupcake pan with paper liners or grease the cups with some butter or cooking spray.
2. In a mixing bowl, beat the butter and sugar until fluffy. Add the eggs, one at a time. Mix well.
3. Mix in the chocolate syrup and vanilla.
4. Mix together the flour and coffee granules.
5. Combine the two mixtures and mix until smooth and without visible lumps.

6.    Evenly distribute the batter among the cups.
7.    Bake for 25–30 minutes until golden brown.
      Check by inserting a toothpick; if it doesn't
      come out clean, bake for a few more minutes
      and repeat.
8.    Leave the pan in the oven for 5 minutes to
      cool slightly.
9.    Remove from oven and let cool on a wire rack
      for 10–15 minutes.
10.   Serve warm.

<u>Ganache</u>
1.    Mix all of the ingredients together. Microwave
      until completely melted. Mix well.
2.    Dip the tops of the cupcakes in the ganache.
3.    Set aside to firm up before serving.

***Nutrition (per serving)***
Calories 407

Carbs 36.5g, Fat 13.4g, Protein 7.1g, Sodium 214mg

# Lemon Cupcakes

*Serves 16*
*Preparation time:15 minutes*
*Cooking time: 20 minutes*

**Ingredients**
3 cups self-rising flour
½ teaspoon salt
½ cup canna-butter, room temperature
½ cup unsalted butter, room temperature
2 cups sugar
4 eggs, room temperature
1 teaspoon vanilla extract
2 tablespoons lemon zest
1 cup whole milk
2½ tablespoons lemon juice

Icing
2 cups heavy cream
¾ cup confectioners' sugar
1½ tablespoons lemon juice

**Directions**
1.  Preheat the oven to 375°F (190°C). Line a
    16-cup muffin or cupcake pan with paper
    liners or grease the cups with some butter or
    cooking spray.
2.  Mix the flour and salt together in a mixing
    bowl.

3. In another mixing bowl, beat both of the butters and the sugar until fluffy. Add the eggs, one at a time, as well as the vanilla and lemon zest. Mix well.
4. Combine the two mixtures and mix until smooth and with no visible lumps. Mix in the lemon juice and milk.
5. Evenly distribute the batter among the cups.
6. Bake for 15–20 minutes until golden brown. Check by inserting a toothpick; if it doesn't come out clean, bake for a few more minutes and repeat.
7. Leave the pan in the oven for 5 minutes to cool slightly.
8. Remove from oven and let cool on a wire rack for 10–15 minutes.
9. Icing:
10. In a mixing bowl, beat the cream and sugar until fluffy. Add half of the lemon juice. Mix well.
11. Add the remaining lemon juice and mix for 5 minutes until soft peaks form.
12. Spread the icing over the cupcakes and serve.


**Nutrition (per serving)**
Calories 384
Carbs 43g, Fat 21g, Protein 4g, Sodium 333mg

# **Blueberry Pie**

*Serves 6-8 slices*
*Preparation time: 10-15 minutes*
*Cooking time: 30-40 minutes*

### Ingredients

2 sheets refrigerated pie crust
1 tablespoon lemon juice
¼ cup all-purpose flour
6 cups fresh or frozen blueberries (or pitted cherries)
½ cup sugar
¼ teaspoon cinnamon
2 tablespoons canna-butter, cut into small pieces

### Directions

1. Preheat the oven to 425°F (220°C). Place one pie crust sheet in a 9-inch pie pan. Press firmly to cover the sides of the pan. The crust should be hanging 1 inch over the edges; trim any excess dough.
2. Mix together the lemon juice, flour, blueberries, sugar and cinnamon.
3. Pour over the pan; add the canna-butter pieces evenly on top.
4. Arrange the second pie crust sheet on top. The crust should be hanging 1 inch over the edges; trim any excess dough.
5. Fold and pinch the edges together to create a seal.
6. Make slits in the top with a knife.
7. Bake for 20 minutes. Reduce temperature to to 350°F (175°C).

8. Bake for 30–40 minutes until the top and edges turn golden brown and the filling is bubbling.
9. Remove from oven and let cool completely on a wire rack.
10. Slice and serve.

**Nutrition (per serving)**
Calories 331
Carbs 47g, Fat 15g, Protein 3g, Sodium 235mg

# Apple Pie

*Serves 6-8 slices*
*Preparation time: 10 minutes*
*Cooking time: 45 minutes*

## Ingredients

2 sheets refrigerated pie crust
5 peeled apples, cored and diced
1 cup brown sugar
½ cup white sugar
1 teaspoon cinnamon
¼ teaspoon nutmeg
1 tablespoon lemon juice
1 teaspoon vanilla extract
1 tablespoon canna-butter
1 egg white

## Directions

1. Preheat the oven to 400°F (200°C). Place one pie crust sheet in a 9-inch pie pan. Press firmly to cover the sides of the pan. The crust should be hanging 1 inch over the edges; trim any excess dough.
2. Add the canna-butter and flour to a medium saucepan or skillet. Heat over medium heat.
3. Add the sugar and all of the spices; stir-cook until simmering.
4. Mix in the lemon juice and vanilla. Stir.
5. Add the apples and stir-cook for 8–10 minutes.

6.   Pour over the pan and arrange the second pie crust sheet on top. The crust should be hanging 1 inch over the edges; trim any excess dough.
7.   Fold and pinch the edges together to create a seal.
8.   Make 4 slits in the top with a knife. Brush egg white on top.
9.   Bake for 45 minutes until the top and edges turn golden brown and the filling is bubbling.
10.  Remove from oven and let cool for 2 hours on a wire rack.
11.  Slice and serve.

**Nutrition (per tablespoon)**
Calories 200
Carbs 51g, Fat 20g, Protein 1g, Sodium 272mg

# Coconut Pie

*Serves Makes 1 pie (8 servings/slices)*
*Preparation time: 10 minutes*
*Cooking time: 40 hours*

### Ingredients
2 cups cannabis milk
1 cup condensed milk
1 (11–12 inch) pie crust
3 large eggs
3 teaspoons vanilla extract
1 cup shredded coconut, lightly toasted
1 cup granulated sugar
½ teaspoon salt
Butter to grease

### Directions
1. Preheat oven to 300°F (148°C)
2. Grease a pie pan with some butter and place the crust in it.
3. Combine the sugar, condensed milk, cannabis milk, eggs, vanilla extract, toasted shredded coconut and salt in a mixing bowl to make a smooth mix.
4. Add the batter to the pie shell and bake for 35–40 minutes or until the pie is well set.
5. Cool down and make slices. Serve warm.

***Nutrition (per serving)***
Calories 523
Carbs 42.3g, Fat 26.8g, Protein 4.6g, Sodium 267mg

# Cherry Pie

*Serves 6–8 slices*
*Preparation time: 25–30 minutes*
*Cooking time: 1 hour*

## Ingredients

2 sheets refrigerated pie crust
½ cup all-purpose flour
4 cups cherries, pitted
1 cup sugar
¼ cup canna-butter
½ teaspoon vanilla extract
1 teaspoon sugar

## Directions

1. Preheat the oven to 375°F (190°C). Place one pie crust sheet in a pie pan. Press firmly to cover the sides of the pan. The crust should be hanging 1 inch over the edges; trim any excess dough.
2. Mix together the flour, cherries, sugar and canna-butter.
3. Mix in the vanilla extract.
4. Add the filling to the pan and arrange the second pie crust sheet on top. The crust should be hanging 1 inch over the edges; trim any excess dough.
5. Fold and pinch the edges together to create a seal.
6. Make 6 slits in the top with a knife.
7. Refrigerate for 20–25 minutes.

8.	Bake for 55–60 minutes until the top and edges turn golden brown and the filling is bubbling.
9.	Remove from oven and let cool completely on a wire rack.
10.	Sprinkle sugar on top and refrigerate for 1 hour before serving.

**Nutrition (per serving)**
Calories 397
Carbs 62g, Fat 17g, Protein 3g, Sodium 234mg

# Cracker Coconut Bars

*Serves 15-20 bars*
*Preparation time: 10 minutes*
*Cooking time: 25 minutes*

### Ingredients

1 cup canna-butter, melted

1 cup graham cracker crumbs

1 can condensed milk

1 cup coconut, shredded

1 cup chocolate chips

### Directions

1. Preheat the oven to 350°F (175°C).
2. Evenly spread the melted canna-butter over the bottom of a 9×13-inch baking pan.
3. Spread the cracker crumbs evenly on top. Press gently to form an even layer.
4. Sprinkle the coconut and then the chocolate chips over the cracker layer.
5. Pour on the condensed milk.
6. Bake for about 25 minutes until the edges turn golden.
7. Let cool slightly.
8. Slice into squares and serve warm.

### Nutrition (per bar)

Calories 209

Carbs 19g, Fat 14g, Protein 2g, Sodium 522mg

# CAKES AND MUFFINS

## Pumpkin Muffins

*Serves 24 muffins*
*Preparation time: 10-15 minutes*
*Cooking time: 25 minutes*

### Ingredients

2½ cups all-purpose flour
1½ teaspoons baking soda
1¼ teaspoons salt
1¼ teaspoons ground cinnamon
1⅛ teaspoons ground nutmeg
¾ teaspoon ground cloves
½ teaspoon ground ginger
3 eggs
1½ cups sugar
3 tablespoons canna-oil
⅓ cup + 2 tablespoons vegetable oil
½ cup water
1 (15-ounce) can pumpkin (*not* pumpkin pie mix)
1 cup walnuts and/or chocolate chips (optional)

### Directions

1. Preheat the oven to 350°F (175°C). Line two 12-cup muffin pans with paper liners or grease the cups with some butter or cooking spray.

2.  Mix the flour, baking soda, salt, nutmeg, cinnamon, cloves and ginger together in a mixing bowl.
3.  In another bowl, beat the eggs. Add the sugar, oils and water. Mix well.
4.  Mix in the pumpkin.
5.  Combine the two mixtures and mix until smooth and without visible lumps.
6.  Mix in the chocolate chips and/or walnuts.
7.  Evenly distribute the batter among the muffin cups.
8.  Bake for 25 minutes until golden brown. Check by inserting a toothpick; if it doesn't come out clean, bake for a few more minutes and repeat.
9.  Leave the pan in the oven for 5 minutes to cool slightly.
10. Remove from oven and let cool on a wire rack for about 10 minutes.
11. Gently remove the muffins from the cups before serving.

### Nutrition (per serving)

Calories 168

Carbs 25g, Fat 6g, Protein 2g, Sodium 212mg

# Banana Cinnamon Muffins

*Serves 10 muffins*
*Preparation time: 10 minutes*
*Cooking time: 20 minutes*

**Ingredients**
1½ cups all-purpose flour
1 teaspoon baking soda
1 teaspoon baking powder
½ teaspoon salt
1 egg, lightly beaten
3 mashed bananas
¾ cup white sugar
⅓ cup canna-butter, melted
⅓ cup packed brown sugar
2 tablespoons all-purpose flour
⅛ teaspoon ground cinnamon
1 tablespoon butter

**Directions**
1. Preheat the oven to 375°F (190°C). Line a 10-cup muffin pan with paper liners or grease the cups with some butter or cooking spray.
2. Mix the 1½ cups of flour, baking soda, baking powder and salt together in a mixing bowl.
3. In another bowl, beat the eggs. Add the bananas, sugar and canna-butter. Mix well.
4. Combine the two mixtures and mix until smooth and without visible lumps.
5. Evenly distribute the batter among the muffin cups.

6.   Mix the brown sugar, 2 tablespoons of flour and cinnamon together in a mixing bowl.
7.   Add the butter and continue to mix until you get coarse, meal-like consistency.
8.   Divide evenly among the muffin cups.
9.   Bake for 20 minutes until golden brown. Check by inserting a toothpick; if it doesn't come out clean, bake for a few more minutes and repeat.
10.  Leave the pan in the oven for 5 minutes to cool slightly.
11.  Remove from oven and let cool on a wire rack for about 10 minutes.
12.  Gently remove the muffins from the cups before serving.

**Nutrition (per serving)**

Calories 263

Carbs 35g, Fat 8g, Protein 3g, Sodium 267mg

# Walnut Zucchini Muffins

*Serves 12 muffins*
*Preparation time: 10 minutes*
*Cooking time: 20 minutes*

### Ingredients
1½ cups zucchini, grated
½ cup canna-butter, melted
¼ cup olive oil
½ cup white sugar
½ cup brown sugar
2 eggs
½ teaspoon baking powder
½ teaspoon baking soda
½ teaspoon salt
¼ teaspoon cinnamon
¼ teaspoon nutmeg
2 cups all-purpose flour
½ cup chopped walnuts (optional)

### Directions
1. Preheat the oven to 350°F (175°C). Line a 12-cup muffin pan with parchment paper liners.
2. Mix the zucchini, canna-butter, olive oil, white sugar and brown sugar together in a mixing bowl.
3. In another bowl, beat the eggs. Add the other dry ingredients. Mix well.
4. Combine the two mixtures and mix until smooth and without visible lumps.

5.   Mix in the nuts, if using.
6.   Evenly distribute the batter among the muffin cups.
7.   Bake for 20 minutes until golden brown. Check by inserting a toothpick; if it doesn't come out clean, bake for a few more minutes and repeat.
8.   Leave the pan in the oven for 5 minutes to cool slightly.
9.   Remove from oven and let cool on a wire rack for about 10 minutes.
10.  Gently remove the muffins from the cups before serving.

### *Nutrition (per serving)*

Calories 290

Carbs 33g, Fat 14g, Protein 4g, Sodium 168mg

# Blueberry Muffins

*Serves 12 muffins*
*Preparation time: 10 minutes*
*Cooking time: 16 minutes*

### Ingredients
1½ cups all-purpose flour
¾ cup sugar
2 teaspoons baking powder
½ teaspoon nutmeg (optional)
¼ teaspoon salt
1 large egg
¼ cup canna-oil
¼ cup coconut oil
⅓ cup milk
1½ teaspoons vanilla extract
1 cup fresh or unthawed frozen blueberries

### Directions
1. Preheat the oven to 300°F (150°C). Line a 12-cup muffin pan with parchment paper liners.
2. Mix the flour, sugar, baking powder, salt and nutmeg together in a mixing bowl.
3. In another bowl, beat the eggs. Add the oil, milk and vanilla. Mix well.
4. Combine the two mixtures and mix until smooth and without visible lumps.
5. Mix in the blueberries.
6. Evenly distribute the batter among the muffin cups. Sprinkle some sugar on top.

7.  Bake for 18 minutes until golden brown. Check by inserting a toothpick; if it doesn't come out clean, bake for a few more minutes and repeat.
8.  Leave the pan in the oven for 5 minutes to cool slightly.
9.  Remove from oven and let cool on a wire rack for about 10 minutes.
10. Gently remove the muffins from the cups before serving.

**Nutrition (per serving)**

Calories 161

Carbs 26g, Fat 5g, Protein 2g, Sodium 136mg

# Chocolate Muffins

*Serves 12–15 muffins*
*Preparation time: 10 minutes*
*Cooking time: 15–18 minutes*

## Ingredients

1⅓ cups flour
2 teaspoons baking powder
¼ teaspoon baking soda
¾ cup unsweetened cocoa powder
¼ teaspoon salt
1½ cups sugar
¼ cup canna-butter or canna-oil
2 large eggs
½ teaspoon vanilla extract
1 cup milk

## Directions

1. Preheat the oven to 350°F (175°C). Line a 12–16 cup muffin pan with paper liners or grease the cups with some butter or cooking spray.
2. Mix the flour, baking powder, baking soda, salt and cocoa powder together in a mixing bowl.
3. In another bowl, beat the canna-butter/canna-oil and sugar. Add the eggs. Mix well.
4. Mix in the vanilla.
5. Combine the two mixtures and mix while adding the milk until smooth and with no visible lumps.

6.  Evenly distribute the batter among the muffin cups.
7.  Bake for 15–18 minutes until golden brown. Check by inserting a toothpick; if it doesn't come out clean, bake for a few more minutes and repeat.
8.  Leave the pan in the oven for 5 minutes to cool slightly.
9.  Remove from oven and let cool on a wire rack for about 10 minutes.
10. Gently remove the muffins from the cups before serving.

**Nutrition (per serving)**

Calories 174

Carbs 30g, Fat 5g, Protein 3g, Sodium 132mg

# Cheddar Jalapeño Muffins

*Serves 12-15*
*Preparation time: 10 minutes*
*Cooking time: 30-35 minutes*

### Ingredients
½ cup all-purpose flour
½ teaspoon salt
1 tablespoon baking powder
½ cup canna-butter
⅓ cup sugar
2 large eggs
8 ounces creamed corn
1 cup sour cream
1 cup grated sharp cheddar cheese
1 teaspoon lemon zest
½ cup chopped jalapeño peppers, seeded
1½ cups yellow cornmeal

### Directions
1. Preheat the oven to 325°F (160°C). Grease a 12–15 cup muffin pan with some butter or cooking spray.
2. Mix the flour, salt and baking powder together in a mixing bowl.
3. In another bowl, beat the canna-butter and sugar. Add the eggs. Mix well.
4. Mix in the creamed corn and sour cream.
5. Combine the two mixtures and mix until smooth and with no visible lumps.

6.   Mix in the cheese, lemon zest, jalapeño peppers and cornmeal until smooth and with no visible lumps.
7.   Evenly distribute the batter among the muffin cups.
8.   Bake for 30–35 minutes until golden brown. Check by inserting a toothpick; if it doesn't come out clean, bake for a few more minutes and repeat.
9.   Leave the pan in the oven for 5 minutes to cool slightly.
10.  Remove from oven and let cool on a wire rack for about 10 minutes.
11.  Gently remove the muffins from the cups before serving.

**Nutrition (per serving)**

Calories 215

Carbs 21g, Fat 13g, Protein 5g, Sodium 301mg

# Banana Chocolate Chip Muffins

*Serves 12 muffins*
*Preparation time: 10 minutes*
*Cooking time: 25 minutes*

## Ingredients

1½ cups all-purpose flour
½ cup white sugar
1½ teaspoons baking powder
¼ teaspoon salt
1 large egg
1¼ cups mashed bananas
¼ cup milk
¼ cup canna-butter
1 teaspoon vanilla extract
¼ cup butter, melted
1 cup chocolate chips
2 tablespoons coarse raw sugar

## Directions

1. Preheat the oven to 350°F (175°C). Line a 12-cup muffin pan with paper liners or grease the cups with some butter or cooking spray.
2. Mix the flour, sugar, baking powder and salt together in a mixing bowl.
3. In another bowl, beat the eggs. Add the mashed bananas, milk and canna-butter. Mix well.
4. Mix in the vanilla and butter.

5. Combine the two mixtures and mix until smooth and without visible lumps.
6. Mix in the chocolate chips.
7. Evenly distribute the batter among the muffin cups. Sprinkle the raw sugar on top.
8. Bake for 25 minutes until golden brown. Check by inserting a toothpick; if it doesn't come out clean, bake for a few more minutes and repeat.
9. Leave the pan in the oven for 5 minutes to cool slightly.
10. Remove from oven and let cool on a wire rack for about 10 minutes.
11. Gently remove the muffins from the cups before serving.

**Nutrition (per serving)**

Calories 283

Carbs 37g, Fat 13g, Protein 4g, Sodium 126mg

# Applesauce Muffins

*Serves 12 muffins*
*Preparation time: 10 minutes*
*Cooking time: 20 minutes*

**Ingredients**

3 eggs
1½ cups applesauce
½ cup canna-butter, room temperature
¾ cup brown sugar, golden
2¼ cups flour
3 teaspoons baking powder
3 teaspoons baking soda
1 teaspoon nutmeg
1 teaspoon salt
¼ cup white sugar

**Directions**

1.   Preheat the oven to 425°F (220°C). Line a 12-cup muffin pan with parchment paper liners.
2.   Mix the flour, baking soda, baking powder and spices together in a mixing bowl.
3.   In another bowl, beat the eggs. Add the applesauce, canna-butter and brown sugar. Mix well.
4.   Combine the two mixtures and mix until smooth and without visible lumps.
5.   Cover bowl and refrigerate for 15 minutes to make the batter moist and dense.
6.   Mix in the white sugar.

7.  Evenly distribute the batter among the muffin cups. Sprinkle some more white sugar on top (optional).
8.  Bake for 7 minutes and reduce heat to to 350°F (175°C).
9.  Bake for 12 minutes until golden brown. Check by inserting a toothpick; if it doesn't come out clean, bake for a few more minutes and repeat.
10.  Leave the pan in the oven for 5 minutes to cool slightly.
11.  Remove from oven and let cool on a wire rack for about 10 minutes.
12.  Gently remove the muffins from the cups before serving.

**Nutrition (per serving)**

Calories 188

Carbs 27g, Fat 9g, Protein 3.5g, Sodium 512mg

# Cherry Chocolate Muffins

*Serves 4 muffins*
*Preparation time: 10 minutes*
*Cooking time: 8-10 minutes*

### Ingredients

3½ ounces black chocolate

1¾ ounces canna-butter

2 eggs

3½ ounces powdered sugar

1¾ ounces flour

4 candied cherries

### Directions

1. Preheat the oven to 356°F (180°C). Grease 4 cups of a 12-cup muffin pan with some butter or cooking spray.
2. Microwave the chocolate and canna-butter for 20–30 seconds until the chocolate melts. Mix well.
3. In another bowl, beat the eggs. Add the sugar. Mix well.
4. Mix in the chocolate mixture.
5. Mix in the flour until smooth and without visible lumps.
6. Evenly distribute the batter among the 4 greased muffin cups.
7. Bake for 8–10 minutes. Check by inserting a toothpick; if it doesn't come out clean, bake for a few more minutes and repeat.
8. Leave the pan in the oven for 5 minutes to cool slightly.

9. Remove from oven and let cool on a wire rack for about 10 minutes.
10. Gently remove the muffins from the cups; top each with a cherry and serve warm.

**Nutrition (per serving)**

Calories 255

Carbs 22g, Fat 13g, Protein 4g, Sodium 91mg

# Pumpkin Spice Muffins

*Serves 12 muffins*
*Preparation time: 10 minutes*
*Cooking time: 25 minutes*

### Ingredients

4 eggs
1 cup white sugar
½ cup packed brown sugar
1¼ cups cooking oil
¼ cup canna-oil
2 teaspoons vanilla extract
1¾ cups pumpkin puree
3 cups all-purpose flour
1 tablespoon ground cinnamon
1 tablespoon pumpkin spice
2 teaspoons baking powder
2 teaspoons baking soda
1 tablespoon orange zest (optional)
Pumpkin seeds to taste

### Directions

1. Preheat the oven to 350°F (175°C). Line a 12-cup muffin pan with parchment paper liners.
2. In another bowl, beat the eggs. Add both of the sugars, cooking oil and canna-oil. Mix well.
3. Mix in the vanilla and pumpkin puree.
4. Mix all of the dry ingredients together in a mixing bowl.

5. Combine the two mixtures and mix until smooth and without visible lumps.
6. Mix in the orange zest, if using.
7. Evenly distribute the batter among the muffin cups. Sprinkle with pumpkin seeds.
8. Bake for 22–25 minutes until golden brown. Check by inserting a toothpick; if it doesn't come out clean, bake for a few more minutes and repeat.
9. Leave the pan in the oven for 5 minutes to cool slightly.
10. Remove from oven and let cool on a wire rack for about 10 minutes.
11. Gently remove the muffins from the cups before serving.

### Nutrition (per serving)

Calories 236

Carbs 45g, Fat 2g, Protein 5g, Sodium 226mg

# Chocolate Spice Cake

*Serves 8–10*
*Preparation time: 10–15 minutes*
*Cooking time: 50–60 minutes*

**Ingredients**

1 cup chopped walnuts
2½ cups sugar (divided)
1 cup chocolate chips
1 tablespoon ground cinnamon
½ teaspoon ground cardamom
1 cup canna-butter, room temperature
2 large eggs, lightly beaten
2 cups sour cream
1 tablespoon vanilla
2 cups all-purpose flour
1 tablespoon baking powder
¼ teaspoon salt

**Directions**

1.  Preheat the oven to 350°F (175°C). Grease a 9×13-inch baking or cake pan with cooking spray.
2.  Mix the walnuts, ½ cup of the sugar, chocolate chips, cinnamon and cardamom together in a mixing bowl.
3.  In another bowl, combine the remaining sugar and canna-butter. Add the eggs. Mix well.
4.  Add the sour cream and vanilla; mix well.
5.  Mix the flour, baking powder and salt together in a mixing bowl.

6. Combine the flour and egg mixtures until just blended and without visible lumps. Do not overmix.
7. Add ⅓ of the batter to the pan. Top with half of the chocolate mixture. Repeat the layers and add the last ⅓ of the batter on top.
8. Smooth the surface with a spatula or spoon.
9. Bake for 50–60 minutes until the edges turn golden brown. Check by inserting a toothpick; if it doesn't come out clean, bake for a few more minutes and repeat.
10. Remove from oven and let cool completely on a wire rack.
11. Slice and serve.

**Nutrition (per serving)**
Calories 583
Carbs 73g, Fat 21g, Protein 8g, Sodium 274mg

# Pineapple Upside Down Cake

*Serves 8–10*
*Preparation time: 10–15 minutes*
*Cooking time: 45 minutes*

**Ingredients**
½ cup butter, melted
½ cup light brown sugar
7 pineapple slices
½ cup maraschino cherries

<u>Cake filling</u>
1½ cups flour
½ teaspoon baking powder
½ teaspoon baking soda
½ teaspoon salt
½ cup canna-butter, melted
½ cup light brown sugar
½ cup white sugar
2 eggs
½ cup milk
½ cup unsweetened pineapple juice
1 teaspoon vanilla extract

**Directions**
1.  Preheat the oven to 350°F (175°C). Grease an 8×8-inch baking or cake pan with the melted butter.

2.  Sprinkle sugar evenly over the greased
    surface.
3.  Arrange the pineapple slices and cherries
    over the bottom.
4.  Mix the flour, baking powder, baking soda
    and salt together in a mixing bowl.
5.  In another bowl, mix the sugars and canna-
    butter until smooth without visible lumps.
6.  Mix in the eggs and whisk well.
7.  Add the milk, pineapple juice and vanilla;
    continue to whisk.
8.  Combine the two mixtures and mix until
    smooth and without visible lumps.
9.  Pour the batter into the pan over the fruit.
10. Bake for 20 minutes. Loosely cover the pan
    with aluminum foil.
11. Bake for 25 more minutes. Check by inserting
    a toothpick; if it doesn't come out clean, bake
    for a few more minutes and repeat.
12. Let cool for about 15–20 minutes.
13. Turn the cake upside down, slice and serve.

**Nutrition (per serving)**
Calories 389
Carbs 49g, Fat 21g, Protein 4g, Sodium 258mg

# Red Velvet Cake

*Serves 8–10*
*Preparation time: 15–20 minutes*
*Cooking time: 30–35 minutes*

### Ingredients
2¾ cups all-purpose flour
1¾ cups sugar
1 teaspoon baking soda
2 teaspoons cocoa powder
2 large eggs, room temperature
¾ canna-oil
¾ cup canola oil
1¼ cups buttermilk
2 teaspoons red food coloring
1 teaspoon vanilla extract
1 tablespoon white vinegar

<u>Frosting</u>
16 ounces cream cheese
½ cup softened butter or canna-butter
3 cups powdered sugar
2 teaspoons vanilla extract

### Directions
1. Preheat the oven to 325°F (160°C). Line an 8×8-inch baking or cake pan with parchment paper.
2. Mix the dry ingredients together in a mixing bowl.

3. In another bowl, beat the eggs. Add the oils, food coloring, buttermilk, white vinegar and vanilla. Mix well.
4. Combine the two mixtures and mix until smooth and without visible lumps.
5. Add the batter to the pan and smooth the surface with a spatula or spoon.
6. Bake for 30–35 minutes until the edges turn golden brown. Check by inserting a toothpick; if it doesn't come out clean, bake for a few more minutes and repeat.
7. Remove from oven and let cool completely on a wire rack.
8. Spread icing over the cake, slice and serve.
9. Icing:
10. Mix the butter and cream cheese.
11. Add the sugar and mix well.
12. Mix in the vanilla.

**Nutrition (per serving)**
Calories 718
Carbs 86g, Fat 31g, Protein 7g, Sodium 283mg

# Chocolate Cupcakes

*Serves 24 cupcakes*
*Preparation time: 10–15 minutes*
*Cooking time: 20 minutes*

**Ingredients**

<u>Cupcakes</u>
½ cup cannabis coconut or cannabis olive oil
2 eggs
1 cup buttermilk
1 cup vegetable oil
1½ cups sugar
1 teaspoon vanilla extract
2½ cups all-purpose flour
⅜ cup cocoa powder
2 teaspoons baking soda
¾ teaspoon salt

<u>Icing</u>
1 teaspoon vanilla extract
8 ounces cream cheese
½ cup unsalted butter, melted
3½ cups confectioners' sugar

**Directions**
1. Preheat oven to 350°F or 176°C. Arrange 24 muffin cups with paper cupcake liners.
2. In a medium-large mixing bowl, thoroughly combine the buttermilk, coconut or cannabis

olive oil, vegetable oil, eggs, and vanilla
extract.
3. Whisk the mixture thoroughly or use an
   immersion blender.
4. In another bowl, stir together the flour, sugar,
   cocoa powder, baking soda, and salt.
5. Whisk the dry and wet mixture and mix just
   until smooth.
6. Pour the batter into the prepared muffin cups;
   fill them ⅔ full.
7. Bake for 18-20 minutes or until a toothpick
   comes out clean.
8. Let cool completely.

<u>Icing</u>
1. Mix together the cream cheese, butter and
   vanilla extract in a mixing bowl using an
   electric mixer until fluffy.
2. Add the sugar and continue mixing until the
   sugar dissolves.
3. Spread the icing over the cupcakes and serve.

**Nutrition (per serving)**
Calories 324
Carbs 35.6g, Fat 16.8g, Protein 3.6g, Sodium 216mg

# Poppy Seed Cream Cake

*Serves 8-10*
*Preparation time: 10 minutes*
*Cooking time: 35-40 minutes*

**Ingredients**
<u>Cake</u>
1¾ cups flour
½ teaspoon baking powder
½ teaspoon baking soda
⅛ teaspoon salt
½ cup unsalted canna-butter, softened
1¼ cups sugar
3 eggs
1 cup crème fraîche
3 tablespoons poppy seeds
½ teaspoon almond extract

<u>Frosting</u>
4 ounces cream cheese, softened
⅔ cup powdered sugar
1 cup crème fraîche
1 teaspoon finely grated lemon peel
⅛ teaspoon almond extract

**Directions**
1.	Preheat the oven to 350°F (175°C). Grease a 9×9-inch baking or cake pan with some cooking spray.

2. Mix the flour, baking powder, baking soda and salt together in a mixing bowl.
3. In another bowl, beat the butter and sugar until fluffy. Add the eggs one by one. Mix well.
4. Add the flour mixture in three parts, mixing after each addition. Add the cream fraîche along with the first portion of flour. Mix until smooth and without visible lumps.
5. Mix in the almond extract and poppy seeds.
6. Add the batter to the pan and smooth the surface with a spatula or spoon.
7. Bake for 35–40 minutes until the edges turn golden brown. Check by inserting a toothpick; if it doesn't come out clean, bake for a few more minutes and repeat.
8. Remove from oven and let cool completely on a wire rack.
9. Spread frosting on top. Slice and serve fresh or refrigerate to serve chilled.
10. Frosting:
11. Beat the sugar and cream cheese in a mixing bowl.
12. Mix in the crème fraîche.
13. Mix in the almond extract and lemon peel.

### *Nutrition (per serving)*

Calories 404

Carbs 47g, Fat 19g, Protein 6g, Sodium 154mg

# Chocolate Space Cake

*Serves 24*
*Preparation time: 10 minutes*
*Cooking time: 35 minutes*

**Ingredients**

2¼ cups all-purpose flour
½ teaspoon salt
2 teaspoons baking soda
½ cup canna-butter
2½ cups packed brown sugar
3 eggs
3 (1-ounce) squares unsweetened chocolate, melted
1½ teaspoons vanilla extract
1 cup sour cream
1 cup boiling water

**Directions**

1. Preheat the oven to 350°F (175°C). Grease a 9×13-inch baking or cake pan with some butter or cooking spray.
2. Mix the flour, baking soda and salt together in a mixing bowl.
3. In another bowl, beat the canna-butter and brown sugar. Add the eggs one by one. Mix well.
4. Mix in the vanilla and melted chocolate.
5. Add half of the flour mixture and ½ cup of the sour cream; mix well.

6.   Add the remaining cream and flour and the boiling water. Mix until smooth and without visible lumps.
7.   Add the batter to the pan and smooth the surface with a spatula or spoon.
8.   Bake for 35 minutes until the edges turn golden brown. Check by inserting a toothpick; if it doesn't come out clean, bake for a few more minutes and repeat.
9.   Remove from oven and let cool completely on a wire rack.
10.   Slice and serve.

### Nutrition (per serving)
Calories 191
Carbs 32g, Fat 6g, Protein 2g, Sodium 196mg

# COOKIES

## Almond Meal Cookies

*Serves 15-20 cookies*
*Preparation time: 10 minutes*
*Baking time: 10-20 minutes*

### Ingredients

8 ounces canna-butter, cold and cubed
1⅓ cups powdered sugar
2 egg yolks
½ teaspoon salt
2½ cups flour
1¼ cups almond meal

### Directions

1. In a mixing bowl, beat the canna-butter and sugar until fluffy. Add the eggs, one at a time, and mix well.
2. Mix the salt, flour and almond meal together in a mixing bowl.
3. Combine the two mixtures to form a dough ball.
4. Place the dough in a Ziploc bag and refrigerate for 30 minutes.
5. Preheat the oven to 350°F (175°C). Line a cookie/baking sheet with parchment paper.
6. Roll the dough over lightly floured surface to make a thick layer.

7.    Using a cookie cutter or round cutter, cut out as many cookies as you can.
8.    Place the cookies on the parchment paper. Bake for 10–15 minutes until golden brown.
9.    Remove from oven and let cool for 5–10 minutes.
10.   Serve fresh or store in an airtight container.

**Nutrition (per serving)**

Calories 176

Carbs 18g, Fat 11g, Protein 3g, Sodium 60mg

# Pecan Oats Cookies

*Serves 24-36 cookies*
*Preparation time: 10 minutes*
*Cooking time: 12-20 minutes*

## Ingredients
2 large eggs

¾ cup canna-butter

2 cups raw sugar

2 teaspoons vanilla extract

1 tablespoons ground nutmeg

1 tablespoons ground cinnamon

2 cups whole wheat flour

½ teaspoons baking soda

1 teaspoon salt

1½ cups raisins

2 cups rolled oats

2 tablespoons water

1 cup chopped pecans

## Directions
1. Preheat the oven to 350°F (175°C). Grease a cookie/baking sheet with some butter or cooking spray.
2. In another bowl, beat the eggs. Add the canna-butter, sugar and vanilla. Mix well.
3. Mix together the spices, flour, baking soda and salt.
4. Combine the two mixtures and mix until smooth and with no visible lumps. Add the raisins, oats, water and pecans.

5.   Mix into a smooth dough with no visible lumps.
6.   Cover and refrigerate for 20 minutes.
7.   Roll the dough into small balls and press them onto the cookie/baking sheet.
8.   Bake for 12–20 minutes until the tops are golden brown.
9.   Remove from oven and let cool for 5–10 minutes.
10.  Serve fresh or store in an airtight container.

### *Nutrition (per tablespoon)*
Calories 148

Carbs 21g, Fat 6g, Protein 2g, Sodium 94mg

# Chocolate Oat Cookies

*Serves 35-45 cookies*
*Preparation time: 10 minutes*
*Cooking time: 10-15 minutes*

**Ingredients**

Dry
2¼ cups all-purpose flour
¼ teaspoon baking soda
½ teaspoon salt
2¼ cups oats

Wet
2 eggs
1 egg white
½ cup canna-butter
½ cup coconut oil
¾ cup palm sugar
¼ cup agave or maple syrup
1 teaspoon vanilla extract

Other
1 cup dark chocolate chips
½ cup chopped nuts

**Directions**

1.	Preheat the oven to 350°F (175°C). Line a baking tray with parchment paper.
2.	Mix the dry ingredients together in a mixing bowl.

3. In another bowl, beat the eggs and egg whites. Add the other wet ingredients. Mix well.
4. Combine the two mixtures and mix until smooth and with no visible lumps.
5. Mix in the chocolate chips and nuts.
6. Drop spoonfuls of the dough over the parchment paper, leaving some space between each.
7. Round up each cookie with the back of a spoon.
8. Bake for 10–15 minutes until the tops are golden brown.
9. Remove from oven and let cool for 5–10 minutes.
10. Serve fresh or store in an airtight container.

**Nutrition (per serving)** (4 ounces)
Calories 105
Carbs 10g, Fat 6g, Protein 2g, Sodium 39mg

# Classic Chocolate Chip Cookies

*Serves 30 cookies*
*Preparation time: 10 minutes*
*Cooking time: 12-15 minutes*

**Ingredients**

¼ cup canna-butter, melted
¼ cup unsalted butter, melted
1 teaspoon vanilla extract
⅔ cup sugar
⅔ cup brown sugar
1 egg
½ teaspoon baking soda
½ teaspoon salt
1 cup + 2 tablespoons all-purpose flour
1 cup chocolate chips
Toasted walnuts, chopped, to taste (optional)

**Directions**

1. Preheat oven to 375°F (190°C).
2. Whisk the sugar, brown sugar, canna-butter, butter and vanilla extract in a mixing bowl until creamy.
3. Beat the egg in another bowl; mix with the butter mixture.
4. Stir together the flour, baking soda and salt in another bowl.

5. Mix the dry ingredients into the butter mixture to combine well.
6. Stir in the chocolate chips and nuts.
7. Drop tablespoons of dough onto 2 ungreased baking sheets; keep 1 inch between each drop.
8. Bake for 12–15 minutes until golden brown.
9. Cool on a wire rack, then serve immediately.

**Nutrition (per serving)**
Calories 122
Carbs 16.3g, Fat 5.2g, Protein 1.5g, Sodium 64mg

# Sesame Seed Cookies

*Serves 24 cookies*
*Preparation time: 5-10 minutes*
*Baking time: 5-8 minutes*

### Ingredients

1 cup palm sugar
2 tablespoons dark agave syrup or maple syrup
8 ounces unsalted canna-butter, room temperature
2 eggs
Pinch of salt
⅛ teaspoon baking powder
1⅓ cups all-purpose flour
2½ cups sesame seeds, toasted

### Directions

1. Preheat the oven to 350°F (175°C). Line a baking tray with parchment paper or grease it with some butter or cooking spray.
2. In a mixing bowl, beat the butter, maple syrup and sugar until fluffy. Add the eggs, one at a time. Mix well.
3. Mix together the salt, baking powder, flour and sesame seeds.
4. Combine the two mixtures and mix until smooth and without visible lumps.
5. Drop spoonfuls of the dough over the baking tray, leaving some space between each.
6. Round up each cookie with the back of a spoon.
7. Bake for 6–8 minutes until the tops are golden brown.

8. Remove from oven and let cool for 5–10 minutes.
9. Serve fresh or store in an airtight container.

**Nutrition (per serving)**
Calories 207
Carbs 13g, Fat 15g, Protein 4g, Sodium 26mg

# Almond Chocolate Cookies

*Serves 10*
*Preparation time: 5–10 minutes*
*Cooking and baking time: 20 minutes*

### Ingredients

2 cups almonds, sliced
3 tablespoons all-purpose flour
1 tablespoon powdered orange zest
¼ teaspoon salt
½ cup sugar
⅛ cup coconut oil
⅛ cup canna-oil
2 tablespoons brown rice syrup
2 tablespoons full-fat coconut milk
1 teaspoon vanilla extract
¼–⅓ cup dark chocolate chips
Powdered sugar (optional)

### Directions

1. Preheat the oven to 300°F (150°C). Line two cookie/baking sheets with parchment paper.
2. Mix the flour, almonds, orange zest, salt and sugar together in a mixing bowl.
3. Add both oils, the rice syrup and coconut milk to a medium saucepan or skillet and heat over medium heat.
4. Remove from heat and mix in the vanilla.
5. Add the flour mixture and mix until smooth and without visible lumps. Let cool for 10 minutes.

6.   Drop spoonfuls of the dough over the cookie/baking sheets, leaving some space between each.
7.   Round up each cookie with the back of a spoon.
8.   Bake for 15–17 minutes until the tops are golden brown, rotating the sheets once during cooking.
9.   Remove from oven and let cool for 5–10 minutes.
10.   Microwave the chocolate chips for 20–30 seconds until melted.
11.   Drizzle the chocolate over the cookies and sprinkle powdered sugar on top.
12.   Serve fresh or store in an airtight container.

**Nutrition (per serving)**

Calories 216

Carbs 21g, Fat 14g, Protein 4g, Sodium 62mg

# **Peanut Butter Cookies**

*Serves 24 cookies*
*Preparation time: 10 minutes*
*Cooking time: 10 minutes*

### *Ingredients*
½ cup canna-oil
¾ cup peanut butter
1 cup coconut sugar or ½ cup white sugar + ½ cup
brown sugar
1 large egg, beaten
1¼ cups all-purpose flour
1 teaspoon baking soda
½ teaspoon salt

### *Directions*
1. Preheat the oven to 350°F (175°C). Line a baking tray with parchment paper or grease it with some butter or cooking spray.
2. In a mixing bowl, beat the canna-oil, peanut butter and sugar until fluffy. Add the egg. Mix well.
3. Mix the flour, baking soda and salt together in a mixing bowl.
4. Combine the two mixtures and mix into a smooth dough with no visible lumps.
5. Roll the dough into small balls and press them onto the baking tray.
6. Flatten the balls with a fork, then turn the fork 90° and flatten again to create a crosshatch pattern.

7. Bake for 10 minutes until the tops are golden brown.
8. Remove from oven and let cool for 5–10 minutes.
9. Serve fresh or store in an airtight container.

**Nutrition (per cookie)**

Calories 129

Carbs 11g, Fat 9g, Protein 2g, Sodium 130mg

# Cranberry Oats Cookies

*Serves 24 cookies*
*Preparation time: 10 minutes*
*Baking time: 10-12 minutes*

### Ingredients

½ cup canna-oil
¾ cup light brown sugar
1 egg, beaten
1 teaspoon vanilla
¾ cup oat flour
1½ cups oats
1 teaspoon baking powder
1½ teaspoons cinnamon
½ teaspoon salt
½ teaspoon ginger
¼ cup cranberries, dried
¼ cup dark chocolate chips

### Directions

1. Preheat the oven to 350°F (175°C). Line a cookie/baking sheet with parchment paper.
2. In a mixing bowl, beat the coconut oil and sugar until fluffy. Add the egg and vanilla. Mix well.
3. Mix the dry ingredients together in a mixing bowl.
4. Combine the two mixtures and mix into a smooth dough with no visible lumps.
5. Mix in the cranberries and chocolate chips.

6.    Roll the dough into small balls and press them onto a cookie/baking sheet.
7.    Refrigerate for 30 minutes.
8.    Bake for 10–12 minutes until the tops are golden brown.
9.    Remove from oven and let cool for 5–10 minutes.
10.   Serve fresh or store in an airtight container.

### Nutrition (per cookie)

Calories 71

Carbs 14g, Fat 1g, Protein 1g, Sodium 75mg

# **Walnut Chocolate Chip Cookies**

*Serves 26 cookies*
*Preparation time: 15 minutes*
*Cooking time: 15 minutes*

### Ingredients

1½ cups all-purpose flour
½ teaspoon baking soda
¼ teaspoon baking powder
1 teaspoon salt
6 tablespoons canna-butter
¾ cup dark brown sugar
½ cup white sugar
1 large egg large
1½ teaspoons vanilla extract
1½ cups chocolate chips
¾ cup toffee chips
¾ cup pecans or walnuts, chopped (optional)

### Directions

1. Preheat the oven to 350°F (175°C). Line two cookie/baking sheets with parchment paper or grease with butter or cooking spray.
2. Mix the flour, baking soda, baking powder and salt together in a mixing bowl.
3. In another mixing bowl, beat the canna-butter and both sugars until fluffy. Add the egg and vanilla. Mix well.

4. Combine the two mixtures and mix into a smooth dough with no visible lumps.
5. Mix in the chocolate chips and nuts.
6. Drop spoonfuls of the dough over the cookie/baking sheets, leaving some space between each.
7. Round up each cookie with the back of a spoon.
8. Bake for 15 minutes until the tops are golden brown.
9. Remove from oven and let cool for 5–10 minutes.
10. Serve fresh or store in an airtight container for up to 4 days.

**Nutrition (per serving)**

Calories 205

Carbs 27g, Fat 10g, Protein 2g, Sodium 144mg

# Mint Chocolate Cookies

*Serves 18 cookies*
*Preparation time: 10 minutes*
*Cooking time: 12 minutes*

### Ingredients
½ cup canna-butter, softened
1 cup sugar
1 egg, beaten
½ teaspoon mint extract
1¼ cups all-purpose flour
½ cup unsweetened cocoa powder
¼ teaspoon salt

<u>Melted Chocolate</u>
3 (1-ounce) pieces semisweet chocolate, chopped
¼ cup canna-butter

### Directions
1. Preheat the oven to 350°F (175°C). Grease two cookie/baking sheets with some butter or cooking spray.
2. In a mixing bowl, beat the canna-butter and sugar until fluffy. Add the egg and mint extract. Mix well.
3. Mix the flour, cocoa and salt together in another mixing bowl.
4. Add the flour mixture to the egg mixture in two batches. Mix into a smooth dough with no visible lumps.

5.  Divide the dough into two parts. Roll each parts over a lightly floured surface to make a 1½-inch diameter cylinder.
6.  Wrap with wax paper and refrigerate for 5 hours.
7.  Remove from refrigerator and set aside for 30 minutes at room temperature.
8.  Slice each roll into ¼-inch-thick pieces.
9.  Arrange the cookies on the baking sheets.
10. Bake for 10–12 minutes until the tops are golden brown.
11. Remove from oven and let cool for 5–10 minutes.
12. Mix the chocolate and canna-butter. Microwave for 20–30 seconds until melted. Mix well.
13. Drizzle the chocolate over the cookies.

***Nutrition (per serving)***
Calories 153
Carbs 19g, Fat 8g, Protein 2g, Sodium 104mg

# Coconut Macaroons

*Serves 25-35 macaroons*
*Preparation time: 10 minutes*
*Baking time: 15–17 minutes*

### Ingredients

¾ cup sugar

2 large egg whites

2 cups shredded coconut

⅔ cup chopped almonds

5 tablespoons + 1 teaspoon canna-oil

2 teaspoons vanilla extract

½ teaspoon almond extract

Pinch of salt

1 cup dark or white chocolate, melted (optional)

### Directions

1. Preheat the oven to 340°F (170°C). Line a cookie/baking sheet with parchment paper.
2. In another bowl, beat the eggs and sugar for 2–3 minutes until fluffy.
3. Mix the coconut, almonds, canna-oil, vanilla and almond extracts, and salt together in a mixing bowl.
4. Combine the two mixtures and mix into a smooth dough with no visible lumps.
5. Drop spoonfuls of dough over the cookie/baking sheet, leaving some space between each.
6. Round up each cookie with the back of a spoon.

7.  Bake for 15–17 minutes until the tops are golden brown.
8.  Remove from oven and let cool for 5–10 minutes.
9.  Drizzle the cookies with melted chocolate, if using.
10. Serve fresh or store in an airtight container.

### *Nutrition (per macaroon)*

Calories 91

Carbs 12g, Fat 3g, Protein 2g, Sodium 36mg

# Classic Sugar Cookies

*Serves 24 cookies*
*Preparation time: 15-20 minutes*
*Cooking time: 10-12 minutes*

### Ingredients

2½ cups all-purpose flour
1 teaspoon baking powder
1 teaspoon salt
1 cup canna-butter
1 cup sugar
1 egg
1 teaspoon vanilla extract

<u>Optional frosting</u>
Milk, powdered sugar, and food coloring of your choice

### Directions

1. Preheat the oven to 375°F (190°C). Line two cookie/baking sheets with parchment paper.
2. Mix the dry ingredients together in a mixing bowl.
3. In another mixing bowl, beat the canna-butter and sugar until fluffy. Add the egg and vanilla. Mix well.
4. Combine the two mixtures and mix into a smooth dough with no visible lumps.
5. Cover and refrigerate for 1 hour.
6. Roll the dough over a lightly floured surface to make a thick layer.

7.    Using a cookie cutter or round cutter, cut out 24 cookies.
8.    Place the cookies on the cookie/baking sheets.
9.    Bake for 10–12 minutes until the tops are golden brown.
10.    Remove from oven and let cool for 5–10 minutes.
11.    To make the optional frosting, beat the milk, sugar and food coloring in a mixing bowl until completely dissolved. Spread the frosting over the cookies.
12.    Serve fresh or store in an airtight container.

**Nutrition (per serving)**
Calories 175

Carbs 23g, Fat 8g, Protein 2g, Sodium 120mg

# White Chocolate Cookies

*Serves 20-24 cookies*
*Preparation time: 10 minutes*
*Cooking time: 12 minutes*

## Ingredients

1 cup canna-oil
¾ cup brown sugar
1 egg
2 tablespoons vanilla extract
1 cup all-purpose flour
½ teaspoon baking powder
½ pound white chocolate, chopped

## Directions

1. Preheat the oven to 360°F (180°C). Line a cookie/baking sheet with parchment paper.
2. In a mixing bowl, beat the canna-oil and sugar until fluffy. Add the egg and vanilla. Mix well.
3. Mix together the flour and baking powder.
4. Combine the two mixtures and mix into a smooth dough with no visible lumps.
5. Mix in the white chocolate.
6. Roll the dough into small balls and press them onto the cookie/baking sheet.
7. Bake for 12 minutes until the tops are golden brown.
8. Remove from oven and let cool for 5–10 minutes.
9. Serve fresh or store in an airtight container.

***Nutrition (per cookie)***
Calories 102
Carbs 16g, Fat 4g, Protein 1g, Sodium 15mg

# Pecan Chocolate Biscotti

*Serves 18–24 pieces*
*Preparation time: 15 minutes*
*Cooking time: 40 minutes*

### Ingredients
1¾ cups all-purpose flour
¼ cup unsweetened cocoa powder
1 teaspoon baking soda
¾ teaspoon salt
¼ cup canna-butter
¼ cup butter
¾ cup sugar
2 large eggs
2 teaspoons vanilla extract
1 cup semisweet chocolate chips
¼ cup chopped pecans
2 tablespoons chopped pitted dates

### Directions
1. Preheat the oven to 340°F (170°C). Line a baking sheet with parchment paper.
2. Mix the flours, cocoa powder, baking soda and salt together in a mixing bowl.
3. In another bowl, beat the eggs.
4. In a mixing bowl, beat both of the butters and the sugar until fluffy. Add the eggs, one at a time, and the vanilla. Mix well.
5. Combine the two mixtures and mix into a smooth dough with no visible lumps.
6. Mix in the chocolate, dates and pecans.

7.   Divide into three portions and roll to make
     three 6-inch logs.
8.   Arrange the logs on the baking sheet. Flatten
     slightly with your hands.
9.   Bake for about 28 minutes.
10.  Let cool for a while and then slice diagonally
     into ½-inch pieces.
11.  Return to the oven. Reduce temperature to
     325°F (160°C). Bake for 6 minutes. Turn
     each log and then bake for 6 minutes more
     until cooked to satisfaction.

***Nutrition (per serving)***
Calories 156
Carbs 21g, Fat 8g, Protein 2g, Sodium 145mg

# No Bake Cookies

*Serves 20–24 cookies*
*Preparation time: 10 minutes*
*Cooking time: 5-8 minutes*

### Ingredients

½ cup canna-butter

½ cup milk

1 cup sugar

⅓ cup cacao powder

1 cup oatmeal

1 cup peanut butter

1 tablespoon vanilla extract

### Directions

1. Heat the canna-butter, milk, sugar and cacao powder in a medium saucepan or skillet over medium heat, stirring occasionally.
2. Mix in the remaining ingredients and keep stirring until heated well.
3. Line a cookie/baking sheet with parchment paper.
4. Pour the mixture over the cookie/baking sheet and spread to make a thick, even layer.
5. Let cool for 10–15 minutes.
6. Slice and serve.

### Nutrition (per cookie)

Calories 141

Carbs 13g, Fat 9g, Protein 3g, Sodium 34mg

# CANNA DESSERT DELIGHTS

## Sticky Buns

*Serves 12*
*Preparation time: 15–20 minutes*
*Cooking time: 45 minutes*

### Ingredients

<u>Dough</u>

3½ cups all-purpose flour

¾ teaspoon salt

¼ cup white sugar

¼ cup canna-butter, melted

1 large egg

1¼ cups milk, warmed to 105°F

2¼ teaspoons instant dry yeast

<u>Gooey Sauce</u>

½ cup canna-butter

1 cup brown sugar

½ cup maple syrup

<u>Cinnamon Sugar</u>

1 cup brown sugar

1½ tablespoons ground cinnamon

¼ cup canna-butter

### Directions

1. To make the dough, mix the flour and salt together in a mixing bowl.
2. In another mixing bowl, beat the butter and sugar until fluffy. Add the egg, milk and yeast. Mix well.
3. Combine the two mixtures and mix into a smooth dough with no visible lumps.
4. Cover and set aside for 2 hours to rise.
5. To make the gooey sauce, mix all of the ingredients together in a mixing bowl.
6. Pour the goo into a 13×9-inch baking pan.
7. Spread evenly and set aside.
8. To make the cinnamon sugar, mix all of the ingredients together in a mixing bowl. Set aside.
9. To assemble, roll the dough into a 12×18-inch rectangle on a lightly floured surface.
10. Spread the cinnamon sugar evenly over the dough. Roll up the dough starting from a long side.
11. Slice with a knife to make 12 pieces.
12. Grease a round baking pan with butter. Pour the gooey sauce at the bottom of the pan.
13. Arrange the dough pieces over the gooey sauce in the baking pan.
14. Cover the pan with a towel; set aside for 1 hour to rise.
15. Preheat the oven to 350°F (175°C). Bake for 40–45 minutes. Let cool for 15 minutes.

### Nutrition (per serving)

Calories 472

Carbs 68g, Fat 15g, Protein 5g, Sodium 163mg

# Caramel Popcorn

*Serves 4*
*Preparation time: 10 minutes*
*Cooking time: 30 minutes*


**Ingredients**
3 quarts (12 cups) popped plain popcorn
⅛ cup canna-butter
¼ cup butter
1 cup dark brown sugar
¼ cup honey
2 teaspoons salt (divided)
¾ teaspoon baking soda
1 teaspoon vanilla extract or maple extract


**Directions**
1. Preheat the oven to 225°F (105°C). Line two cookie/baking sheets with parchment paper or grease with butter or cooking spray.
2. Add the sugars and both butters to a medium saucepan or skillet. Stir well.
3. Mix in the honey and ½ teaspoon of the salt; heat over medium heat until boiling and the sugar dissolves completely.
4. Remove from heat; mix in the baking soda and vanilla/maple extract.
5. Pour over the popcorn and stir to coat evenly.
6. Arrange the popcorn on the cookie/baking sheets and sprinkle with the remaining salt.
7. Bake for 15 minutes. Stir the popcorn gently to break up any clumps.
8. Bake for 15 more minutes.

9.  Let cool before serving. Store in an airtight
    container for up to a week.

**Nutrition (per serving)**
Calories 498
Carbs 88g, Fat 13g, Protein 4g, Sodium 985mg

# Pecan Sandies

*Serves 24 sandies*
*Preparation time: 10 minutes*
*Cooking time: 20 minutes*

### Ingredients

1 cup ground pecans
1 cup canna-butter
2 cups all-purpose flour
½ teaspoon baking powder
1 tablespoon vanilla extract
1 cup brown sugar
2 teaspoons cinnamon
½ cup powdered sugar, sifted

### Directions

1. Preheat the oven to 325°F (160°C).
2. In a mixing bowl, beat the canna-butter and sugar until fluffy. Mix in the vanilla.
3. Mix together the flour and baking powder.
4. Combine the two mixtures and mix until smooth and with no visible lumps. Add the pecans.
5. Cover and refrigerate for 3–4 hours.
6. Make golf-ball-size balls from the dough and place them on an ungreased cookie/baking sheet.
7. Bake for 20 minutes until golden and firm.
8. Let cool for a while, sprinkle with cinnamon and powdered sugar, and serve warm.

**Nutrition (per sandy)**
Calories 182
Carbs 20g, Fat 11g, Protein 1g, Sodium 16mg

# Mini Peach Cobbler

*Serves 12 mini cobblers*
*Preparation time: 15-20 minutes*
*Cooking time: 45 minutes*

### Ingredients

¾ cup diced peaches
1 cup all-purpose flour
1 cup + 3 tablespoons sugar
½ teaspoon cinnamon
¼ teaspoon salt
1½ teaspoons baking powder
½ teaspoon nutmeg
1 cup milk
¼ cup canna-butter, melted
¼ cup unsalted butter, melted
1 teaspoon vanilla extract
Whipped cream, to serve (optional)
Cooking spray to grease

### Directions

1. Preheat oven to 350°F (175°C). Grease 12 muffin tins with some cooking spray.
2. In a mixing bowl, mix the peaches, 3 tablespoons of sugar, and the cinnamon. Set the mixture aside.
3. In a mixing bowl, mix the flour, baking powder, 1 cup of sugar, nutmeg and salt.
4. Whisk in the milk, canna-butter, butter and vanilla extract.

5. Fill each muffin tin about half full and add the
   peach mixture on top.
6. Bake for 40–45 minutes until golden brown.
7. Let cool and serve.

**Nutrition (per serving)**
Calories 193
Carbs 24.6g, Fat 7.6g, Protein 2.7g, Sodium 63mg

# Choco Chip Truffles

*Serves Around 30-35 truffles*
*Preparation time: 20-30 minutes*
*Cooking time: 5 minutes*

## Ingredients

½ cup canna-butter, room temperature
½ cup packed light brown sugar
¼ cup white sugar
2 tablespoons cream or milk
½ teaspoon vanilla extract
1¼ cups all-purpose flour
½ teaspoon salt
½ cup semisweet mini chocolate chips

## Coating

8 ounces dark chocolate candy coating

## Directions

1. Line two baking sheets with parchment paper.
2. In a mixing bowl, beat the butter and both sugar until fluffy. Add the milk and vanilla. Mix well.
3. Mix in the flour and salt until you get a smooth mixture.
4. Mix in the chocolate chips.
5. Cover and refrigerate for 30 minutes until firm.
6. Make 1-inch balls from the dough and place them on the baking sheets.
7. Refrigerate for 10–15 minutes more.

8.	Microwave the chocolate candy coating until completely melted.
9.	Coat the balls evenly with melted chocolate.
10.	Place them on the baking sheets and set aside to firm up.
11.	If you have any leftover coating, you can drizzle it over the truffles with a fork to create a nice finishing touch.

**Nutrition (per truffle)**
Calories 104
Carbs 14g, Fat 5g, Protein 0.5g, Sodium 34mg

# Chocolate Fudge

*Serves 2-4*
*Preparation time: 10-15 minutes*
*Cooking time: 5 minutes*

### Ingredients

2–4 scoops vanilla ice cream
½ teaspoon vanilla extract
¼ cup whipped cream
¼ cup cocoa powder
Chopped nuts, to serve
½ cup corn syrup
¼ cup brown sugar
8 ounces semisweet chocolate chips
1 tablespoon canna-butter

### Directions

1. To a medium skillet or saucepan, add the whipping cream, cocoa, brown sugar and corn syrup; heat over low-medium heat.
2. Let the mixture cool down.
3. Add the canna-butter, vanilla extract and chocolate; combine well to make a smooth mixture.
4. Scoop the ice cream into serving dishes; top with chocolate syrup and chopped nuts.

### Nutrition (per serving)

Calories 568
Carbs 42.6g, Fat 17.6g, Protein 4.6g, Sodium 49mg

# **Peanut Butter Fudge**

*Serves 64 pieces*
*Preparation time: 10-15 minutes*
*Cooking time: 5 minutes*

### Ingredients
1¼ cups canna-butter
1 pound powdered sugar
1½ cups creamy peanut butter
½ teaspoon salt
1½ teaspoons vanilla extract

### Directions
1. Add the canna-butter and peanut butter to a medium saucepan or skillet and heat over medium heat for 4–5 minutes until bubbly.
2. Mix in the vanilla and salt. Remove from heat.
3. Add the powdered sugar and mix until the sugar is dissolved completely and the mixture is smooth.
4. Line an 8×8-inch baking pan with parchment paper.
5. Pour the mixture into the pan and spread evenly.
6. Cover and refrigerate for 1–3 hours.
7. Slice into squares and serve.

### Nutrition (per serving)
Calories 95
Carbs 8.5g, Fat 6.5g, Protein 1.5g, Sodium 43mg

# Strawberry Popsicles

*Serves 6*
*Preparation time: 4-5 hours*
*Cooking time: 0 minutes*

## Ingredients

1¼ cups canna-butter
1 pound powdered sugar
1½ cups creamy peanut butter
½ teaspoon salt
1½ teaspoons vanilla extract

## Directions

1. In a medium-large mixing bowl, thoroughly combine the pureed strawberries, cannabis milk, sugar, yogurt and vanilla extract.
2. Add the diced peaches and transfer the mixture into 6 popsicle molds.
3. Place in the freezer for 4 hours; take out and enjoy.

## Nutrition (per serving)

Calories 46
Carbs 8.6g, Fat 0.3g, Protein 1g, Sodium 19mg

# Flax Fusion Balls

*Serves 4-5*
*Preparation time: 10-15 minutes*
*Cooking time: 0 minutes*

### Ingredients

1 cup dates
1 cup raw almonds
1 cup raw walnuts
2 tablespoons canna-oil or canna-butter
1 tablespoon flax meal
1 tablespoon water
Shredded coconut to taste

### Directions

1. Blend all of the ingredients except for the coconut in a blender or food processor to form a smooth dough. (You can also combine them in a bowl with your hands.)
2. Make golf-ball-size balls from the dough.
3. Add the shredded coconut to a plate. Roll the balls in it to coat them evenly.
4. Store in an airtight container for up to 7 days at room temperature and up to 3 months in the freezer.

### Nutrition (per serving)

Calories 368
Carbs 24g, Fat 21g, Protein 9g, Sodium 32mg

# Caramel Apple Dessert

*Serves 6-8*
*Preparation time: 10 minutes*
*Cooking time: 8-10 minutes*

### Ingredients

½ cup corn syrup
⅓ cup unsalted butter
¾ cup brown sugar
¾ cup sugar
1 tablespoon canna-butter
½ teaspoon salt
⅔ cup heavy whipping cream
4 large apples, peeled and sliced

### Directions

1. To a medium skillet or saucepan, add the brown and white sugars, corn syrup, butter, canna-butter and salt and heat over medium heat.
2. Cook while stirring for 5 minutes to boil the mixture.
3. Lower heat to low and simmer for 2 more minutes.
4. Remove the pan from the heat and stir in the cream.
5. Top the apple slices with the caramel sauce; serve.

**Nutrition (per serving)**
Calories 453
Carbs 34.7g, Fat 14.6g, Protein 1.3g, Sodium 178mg

# Peanut Butter Marshmallow Lips

*Serves 6*
*Preparation time: 10 minutes*
*Cooking time: 0 minutes*

## Ingredients

¼ cup peanut butter
12 apple wedges
Juice of ½ lime
2 tablespoons cannabis coconut or cannabis olive oil
30 small marshmallows

## Directions

1. Top the apple wedges with lime juice.
2. In a mixing bowl, mix the peanut butter and cannabis coconut or cannabis olive oil.
3. Spread the mixture over one side of each apple wedge (not both sides).
4. Add 5 marshmallows to each spread side.
5. Place another wedge on top, with the spread side touching the marshmallows to create a lip-like appearance.
6. Repeat the same with remaining wedges.

## Nutrition (per serving)

Calories 214
Carbs 34.8g, Fat 5.2g, Protein 4.1g, Sodium 66mg

# APPENDIX
## Cooking Conversion Charts

### 1. Measuring Equivalent Chart

| Type | Imperial | Imperial | Metric |
|---|---|---|---|
| Weight | 1 dry ounce | | 28 g |
| | 1 pound | 16 dry ounces | 0.45 kg |
| Volume | 1 teaspoon | | 5 ml |
| | 1 dessert spoon | 2 teaspoons | 10 ml |
| | 1 tablespoon | 3 teaspoons | 15 ml |
| | 1 Australian tablespoon | 4 teaspoons | 20 ml |
| | 1 fluid ounce | 2 tablespoons | 30 ml |
| | 1 cup | 16 tablespoons | 240 ml |
| | 1 cup | 8 fluid ounces | 240 ml |
| | 1 pint | 2 cups | 470 ml |
| | 1 quart | 2 pints | 0.95 l |
| | 1 gallon | 4 quarts | 3.8 l |
| Length | 1 inch | | 2.54 cm |

* Numbers are rounded to the closest equivalent

# 2. Oven Temperature Equivalent Chart

| Fahrenheit (°F) | Celsius (°C) | Gas Mark |
|---|---|---|
| 220 | 100 | |
| 225 | 110 | 1/4 |
| 250 | 120 | 1/2 |
| 275 | 140 | 1 |
| 300 | 150 | 2 |
| 325 | 160 | 3 |
| 350 | 180 | 4 |
| 375 | 190 | 5 |
| 400 | 200 | 6 |
| 425 | 220 | 7 |
| 450 | 230 | 8 |
| 475 | 250 | 9 |
| 500 | 260 | |

* Celsius (°C) = T (°F)-32] * 5/9

** Fahrenheit (°F) = T (°C) * 9/5 + 32

*** Numbers are rounded to the closest equivalent